SPECIAL DIET COOKBOOKS
WHEAT, MILK & EGG-FREE COOKING

Contains delicious and practical recipes for those who need to have these three most common allergens excluded from their diet, as well as information and practical advice on how to cope easily with what seems to be an impossible diet.

SPECIAL DIET COOKBOOKS
WHEAT, MILK & EGG-FREE COOKING

Rita Greer

Thorsons
An Imprint of HarperCollins*Publishers*

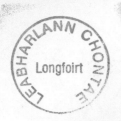
Thorsons
An Imprint of HarperCollins*Publishers*
77-85 Fulham Palace Road,
Hammersmith, London W6 8JB

Illustrations by the author

Published by Thorsons 1984
Second edition 1989
5 7 9 10 8 6 4

A CIP catalogue record for this book
is available from the British Library

ISBN 0-7225-2202-9

Printed and bound in Great Britain by
Hartnolls Ltd, Bodmin, Cornwall

CONTENTS

INTRODUCTION

Wheat, milk and eggs are probably the three most common allergens (allergy-causing agents) in the Western diet today. They are 'staples' and are eaten every day by most of us in some form. While some people may be allergic to just one of these items, others less fortunate may be allergic to all three. As they play such an important part in the structure of our diet, a food regime which excludes them needs to be carefully balanced to replace their valuable nutrients.

The author has had personal and practical experience of catering for a special diet which cuts out wheat, milk and eggs, and the results of her research in the form of information and recipes has proved to be a lifeline for people on similar diets. This book gives a broad outline of the problem of cooking without these foods, and it offers practical advice, including a wide range of recipes, on how to cope with what may at first appear to be an impossible diet to follow.

1.

WHEAT

For most people wheat is a wonderful food! It is cheap, easy to grow and harvest, is highly nutritious and extremely versatile, keeps well and tastes good. One of its most interesting qualities is that when liquid is added to wheat flour it will make a very elastic dough that can be shaped and baked. It will also thicken, make smooth and bind other ingredients. We eat wheat mainly in the form of bread and other bakery products. It is also widely used in a variety of products from instant desserts to toothpaste.

If you see one of the following items listed as an ingredient in a manufactured food, then it may well contain wheat and should be avoided.

Wholewheat or wholegrain	Rusk
Wheat and wheat flour	Wheat germ
Wheat starch	Wheat bran or bran
Wheat protein	Flour
Edible starch	Starch
Food starch	Thickening
Special gluten-free food starch*	Cornflour (cornstarch)

*This is usually wheat starch in disguise.

Contamination by Wheat

Rye, barley, oats and rice are traditionally stored, milled and packed in the same factories and mills as wheat. Contamination is inevitable, as in any flour mill wheat dust is everywhere — all over the machinery, on all ledges and surfaces, on the workers and in the air. So, while it would seem to be the obvious choice to use rye, barley, oats and rice flour on a wheat-free diet the contamination problem has made this impracticable. There is also the point to be considered that rye, barley, oats and rice are not as versatile as wheat for baking, and usually they need to be combined with wheat flour for best results. Oats can be used on their own in a limited way, but appear in the shops as 'rolled oats' and 'oatmeal' and not as a flour. Oats have a very strong taste and are not as bland as wheat.

A very allergic person would be wise not to use rye, barley or rice flour, oats or oatmeal because of the risk of wheat contamination. It is possible to buy ground rice that is guaranteed non-contaminated, but not rice flour. The less allergic person may be able to tolerate the wheat contamination in ordinary milled rye, barley, oats and rice. However, a return of symptoms may mean a stricter approach is necessary, and most people will probably feel it is not worth the risk, preferring a wheat-free diet to a low-wheat diet.

Contamination in the Home

One of the problems of wheat-free baking is that contamination of wheat-free foods and ingredients can occur easily if care is not taken to avoid the problem. The main culprit will be wheat flour which is inclined to be dusty and easily becomes airborne. Wheat may also be present on tins and utensils and this too can lead to contamination. Most people on a wheat-free diet prefer to keep one set of utensils and baking tins etc., just for wheat-free cooking. Wheat flour under the fingernails, wheat flour on overalls or apron can also be a source of contamination. An electric toaster which is used for both wheat bread and wheat-free bread can again be a problem as the crumbs from both kinds of bread accumulate in the bottom. A way round this is to use the grill for toasting wheat-free bread and the toaster for ordinary bread.

For someone who is acutely allergic to wheat a separate set of utensils is a must. Otherwise be scrupulously clean and use the same utensils etc., for both types of baking/cooking.

What Wheat Provides

Basically wheat contributes carbohydrate, protein, vitamins (especially from the B group), minerals (especially iron) and cereal fibre to the diet. In the average diet wheat can provide up to one sixth of the daily intake of protein, more often than not in the form of bread.

To replace wheat in the diet other foods can be used, e.g. protein is readily available in meat and fish. The B-group vitamins can be supplemented by Brewer's Yeast or by vitamin tablets. Many previously bought ready-made foods will need to be made at home, such as bread, cakes, biscuits, etc. If wheat bran has previously been used in the diet, other types of fibre will have to be substituted such as rice bran or soya bran.

What to Avoid

The following other products must not be used in wheat-free cooking *unless you are sure they do not contain any wheat:*

Baked beans in tomato sauce
Baking powder
Batter mixes
Bedtime drinks
Blancmange powders
Biscuits and biscuit mixes
Breadcrumbs
Breakfast cereals
Cakes and cake mixes
Cereals
Chocolate (cheap brands)
Chutney
Cocoa
Coffee (instant)
Cornflour (cornstarch)
Crispbreads
Crumble topping mix
Curry powder
Custard (powder or ready-made tinned)
Gravy powder and mixes
Ice creams
Macaroni
Mustard
Oat porridge
Oatmeal
Pancake mixes
Pastry mixes
Pastas
Pickles
Pie fillings
Porridge
Salad dressings
Sandwich spreads
Sauces
Sausages
Soups (tins and packets)
Soy sauce
Spaghetti
Stock cubes

Desserts and instant puddings   Yogurt (fruit flavours)
Drinking chocolate

2.

MILK

Milk features in our diet in many forms — butter, cream, cheese and yogurt, or as a drink in various ways. In the Western world dairy farming is an extremely important industry and milk is plentiful and cheap. It is not unusual for adults to drink at least one pint (½ litre) per day and children more.

Milk is added to products to enrich them. Components of milk can also be used in manufacturing. Lactose (milk sugar) is widely used as a filler in the manufacture of pharmaceuticals. Caseinate (milk protein) is valuable as an enricher and is used to increase the nutritional value of slimming products and cheeses. Whey is used in the manufacture of margarines usually to make them creamy.

If you see any of the following items listed as an ingredient in a food it will not be milk-free:

Milk	Albumin
Milk solids	Casein
Lactose (milk sugar)	Sodium
Lactic acid	Calcium
Whey	Potassium
Curds	Magnesium } caseinates
Milk protein	Zinc
	Iron

The following products should not be used in milk-free cooking *unless you are sure they do not contain milk:*

Cheeses (all kinds)
Cream
Butter
Margarine
Yogurt
Skimmed milk
Whole milk
Dried milk
Evaporated milk
Condensed milk
Cake mixes
Instant pudding mixes
Pancake and waffle mixes
Creamed foods
Chocolate
Junket
Salad dressings
Yorkshire pudding
Mashed potato

Butter and cream sauces
Instant desserts
Scrambled eggs
Bakery foods, such as cakes,
  buns, pastries and biscuits
Baking powder
Pastry
Chocolate
Sweets
Custard (ready-made)
Slimming foods
Ice cream
Cake toppings
Spreads
Batter mixes
Soups
Chocolate and other milk-
  based drinks

What Milk Provides

Milk contributes carbohydrate, fat, protein, calcium, iron, Vitamin A, Vitamin B_2 and other vitamins and minerals to our diet. It is a liquid food and therefore easy to add to food intake, and it will also mix into other foods easily. To replace milk in the diet other carbohydrate, fat and protein foods such as potatoes, cooking oil, meat and fish can be substituted. Cod liver oil or fish oils will provide Vitamin A. For Vitamin B_2 (Riboflavin) liver is a good source. Calcium can be replaced by Calcium gluconate, Dolomite, B_{13} Calcium (calcium orotate) or bonemeal taken as a supplement. This calcium supplementation is especially important in children's diets as it is necessary for the growth of strong bones, teeth and nails.

Contamination in the Home

Scrupulous cleanliness is essential to avoid contamination, with extra care during washing up. Avoid using the same spoon to stir a non-milk drink when everyone else in the family is having a drink containing milk. This kind of attitude should not be considered to be fussy — merely careful.

Generally speaking milk contamination is less of a hazard than wheat, as milk is usually liquid. Do be careful with dried milk before you mix it with water as it can be dusty and has a nasty habit of sticking to the spoon.

3.
EGGS

Eggs provide a cheap form of food which is very nutritious. Because of the two parts of an egg, the protein-rich white (albumen) and the fat-rich yolk, its versatility in cooking is quite staggering. In particular the white can be aerated to make meringue, and beaten into other foods to bind them together. The yolk can be used to make emulsions such as mayonnaise.

If you see any of the following items listed as an ingredient in a manufactured food it means that egg has been used in its production, and it should therefore be avoided:

Egg	Egg Yolk
Whole egg	Albumen
Dried egg	Egg lecithin
Egg white	Lecithin (unless from soya)

The following must not be used in egg-free cooking, *unless you are sure they do not contain egg:*

Whole egg	Beefburgers
Fresh egg	Fish cakes
Egg yolk	Meat balls
Egg white	Quiche
Dried egg	Scotch egg
Batter mixes	Spaghetti
Sponge and cake mixes	Ice cream
Custard	Bedtime drinks

Salad cream
Mayonnaise
Batter-coated foods (such as
   fish fingers)

Noodles
Sauces
Meringues
Pastas

What Eggs Provide

Eggs contribute protein and fat, calcium, iron, Vitamin A and other vitamins and minerals. They can be replaced in the diet with more meat and fish, but as an aid to cooking they are irreplaceable. You may come across so-called 'egg replacers' while shopping, but a glance at the ingredients list on the pack will reveal that they are largely starch in composition and nutritionally nothing like an egg. However, binders such as grated apple, pectin and methylcellulose can be incorporated into foods so that they don't fall into crumbs. Oils can be substituted for egg yolks to make mayonnaise, but they will not have the yellow colouring of egg yolk.

Contamination in the Home

Extra care is required during cleaning of utensils, cutlery, etc., to avoid contamination. In particular, forks can trap cooked egg between the prongs. Egg white has a very strong tendency to attach itself to utensils, baking sheets, etc. If very stubborn it should be scraped off with a knife. As with wheat and milk contamination the answer to egg contamination is scrupulous cleanliness and great care.

4.

PLANNING A DIET WITHOUT WHEAT, MILK AND EGGS

Before the miseries set in, here is a list of the foods that you can eat:

Basic Wheat-free, Milk-free and Egg-free Foods

Plain, fresh meat (all kinds)
Plain, fresh fish (all kinds)
All fresh vegetables
All fresh fruit
Rice (preferably brown)
Maize (corn)
Plain, fresh nuts
Pure cooking oils, such as safflower, sunflower, soya and corn oils
All kinds of sugar (preferably raw cane) and jams
Bacon

Ham (without breadcrumb coating)
Treacle, syrup and molasses
Pure honey

Drinks:
Wine (red, white or rosé made from fruit)
Brandies derived from fruit
Tea }
Coffee } without milk
Sherry
Port

Other Wheat-free, Milk-free and Egg-free Foods

N.B. Where brand names are specified this indicates that other brands of the same product may be unsuitable.

Baked beans (*Heinz*) in tomato sauce
Soya sauce (*Vesta* or *La Choy*) or any suitable thin soya sauce which is wheat-free
Yeast extract (*Marmite*) or

Split pea flour (yellow)
Soya flour
Ground almonds
Frozen, plain fish and shellfish
Frozen, plain meat
Trufree flours

others made without wheat
Pectin (dried)
Rice bran, soya bran
Soya milk (not to everyone's
taste, but some people find
it useful)
Pulses (split peas, dried beans,
lentils, soya beans)

Trufree crispbran (toasted soya
bran)
Ground rice (preferably
brown)
Curry powder (*Sainsburys,
Vencat UK*) or a brand that
does not contain wheat flour
Gelatine

£22,543/ 641.5631.

Many people find a new kind of diet extremely worrying,
particularly if their basic knowledge of nutrition is not adequate to
restructure their daily menus. To exclude wheat, milk and eggs from
the food regime and still eat a balanced diet can be nutritionally
disastrous if care is not taken over the following points.

The greatest danger lies in eating too little protein, fibre, Vitamin
A, iron and calcium. This can result in a rather alarming weight loss,
constipation, lethargy and a feeling of being 'below par'. Such a
situation is easily rectified by increasing the consumption of fish and
meat, taking a new kind of fibre in the form of rice or soya bran, and
supplementation of the diet with Vitamin A, iron and calcium in
capsule or tablet form. Alternatively, suitable foods that contain these
last three substances can be eaten regularly:

Vitamin A — oily fish;
Iron — curry powder, spinach, watercress, dates, pineapple,
sultanas, cocoa, prunes, figs;
Calcium — sardines, watercress, figs, rhubarb, almonds and
other nuts.

By eating a wide variety of raw or lightly cooked vegetables and
other permitted foods, any other resulting deficiencies in vitamins
and minerals can be made up.

Once the new diet is underway, some people may experience a
craving for wheat, milk and eggs. This is not an unusual reaction
and to cope with it best requires a little extra effort in the kitchen
to make the new diet exciting, satisfying and nutritious.

A Balanced Diet

Nobody knows exactly what each person requires in the way of nutrients as no two people have the same dietary needs. Much depends on what kind of life the person leads, how much energy he or she expends, his or her age and sex.

The average Western diet has many faults — usually containing too much fat, sugar and salt and not enough fibre, fresh vegetables and fruit, because too many processed and 'junk' foods are consumed instead, often merely as a kind of entertainment.

Try to balance the daily food intake in this way:

15 per cent milk-free margarine, nuts, seeds and oils
25 per cent fish and meat
45 per cent fresh fruit and vegetables
15 per cent special bakery items

Try to use plain, fresh foods and not processed ones to minimize problems. The food in a wheat-free, milk-free, egg-free diet is not balanced in the same way as in a diet where these are staples. Here are the basic food values in a wheat-free, milk-free, egg-free diet:

PROTEIN: meat, fish, nuts.
FAT: cooking oils, meat, fish, nuts and seeds.
CARBOHYDRATE: rice, potatoes, bananas, special bread and bakery items, sugar, honey.
FIBRE: soya bran, rice bran, root vegetables, dried fruits.
VITAMINS AND MINERALS: fresh vegetables and fruit.

Bear in mind the advice given at the beginning of this book on replacing the nutrients that will be missing by the exclusion of wheat, milk and eggs. If the need for a vitamin and mineral supplement is felt, remember that like the food, any tablets etc. should also be wheat, milk and egg-free. (See *Useful Information* for information on suppliers.)

Eating Out

Eating out can be a big problem. Most restaurants will be totally unable to cope with a special diet of any description. The safest choice on this particular diet is:

Melon (plain) or fresh grapefruit (plain).
Grilled steak (without gravy or sauce) with a green salad (without dressing).
Fresh fruit.

A word of warning about the use of pepper. It is common practice in commercial catering to add wheat flour to ground white pepper to 'stretch' this expensive commodity. It is therefore a good practice to use only freshly ground black pepper when you are eating out.

Eating out in someone else's home can also be difficult. The majority of hosts/hostesses will not be able to cope with such a strict diet any more than a restaurant can. Many won't want to be bothered to cater for a dieter anyway and will be much relieved when you offer to bring your own food, saving them the trouble of preparing a separate menu and the dieter the worry of eating the wrong things.

The easiest items to take are (for a 3 course meal):

1. Special soup, hot, in a thermos flask, ready to serve;
2. Cold meat, salad and cold, sliced, boiled potatoes — take special dressing in a separate container — arrange on a plate and cover with plastic film until it is served;
3. Fruit salad or fruit, special cheese and crispbreads.

Packed Meals

If meals have to be eaten regularly away from home, packed meals are the answer. Try to balance the meals as you would those eaten at home. Avoid too many snack items which will give you too much carbohydrate.

The easiest items will be hot soup in a vacuum flask; cold meat or canned fish in oil or water; salad with dressing packed in a separate container; crispbreads, cold brown rice or cold potato and fresh fruit and/or a piece of special fruit cake/biscuits. Wide-necked vacuum flasks can be used to take hot meals such as curry and brown rice.

Holidays

Holidays are really just an extension of the eating-out problem. Self-catering holidays, although they are more work, certainly are less worry. Some items such as fruit cake and special bread can be made in advance and taken on holiday to use as required. Any special items that you may have difficulty in obtaining when you get to your destination, such as milk-free margarine, wheat-free soy sauce, special supplements, special brands, etc. must be taken as luggage. With a few exceptions, fresh vegetables, fruit, meat and fish are obtainable everywhere the world over.

Obviously, more planning is needed than for an ordinary holiday and more luggage is needed too. However, there is no reason why holidays away from home shouldn't be enjoyed. If you are travelling by plane take your own packed meal to eat during the flight. If going by car take a picnic, and so on.

If you are on a diet that will make you healthier then that diet is an enviable one. With a little effort your food can be enviable too.

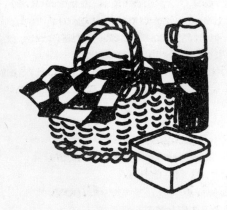

5.

SHOPPING AND THE STORE CUPBOARD

You will find that a special diet needs special shopping, and unless you plan sensibly this could mean extra hours of trekking round the shops without much success. Your best friend in this project could turn out to be the telephone as this will save a tremendous amount of time and energy. Items which you cannot obtain easily may have to be bought by mail order. However you obtain these special foods it is common sense to build up a stock of them in your store cupboard.

Although friends may at first offer assistance with your special shopping they usually become less anxious to help as it starts to become a weekly burden. Usually small shops are more helpful than large stores and will order in say a dozen bottles of a particular kind of soy sauce for you providing you will buy all twelve at once. Although a more expensive way of shopping is to order items by mail it is relatively effortless and they can be delivered right to your door. Usually the more you buy the cheaper it works out, and some firms offer free delivery over a certain amount.

Here is a list of items that could form the basis of a sensible store cupboard and are ones you would be wise not to run out of:

Item	Buy at
Tinned fish in oil — sardines, tuna, salmon	Grocers
Wheat-free thin soy sauce such as *Vesta* or *La Choy* UK	Grocers
Baked beans in tomato sauce (*Heinz* UK)	Grocers

Rice (preferably brown)	Grocers
Ground rice (preferably brown)	Grocers or Health Store
Yellow split pea flour	Health Store or Mail Order
Soya flour	Health Store or Mail Order
Dried pectin	Health Store or Mail Order
Maize flour/cornmeal (make sure of a wheat-free brand)	Grocers
Potato flour	Health Store
Trufree crispbran	Health Store or Mail Order
Vinegar (wine or cider)	Health Store or Grocers
Dried yeast granules	Grocers or Bakers
Gelatine	Grocers
Brown sugar (raw cane)	Health Store or Grocers
Trufree (wheat-free) flours	Health Store or Grocers
Treacle/molasses	Grocers
Salt (sea salt)	Health Store or Grocers
Peppercorns (black)	Grocers
Fruit juices (tinned)	Grocers
Spices (make sure wheat-free brands)	Grocers
Curry powder (make sure wheat-free brands)	Grocers
Dried herbs	Health Store or Grocers

The shops you will use most on this diet are the butcher, fishmonger and greengrocer, so most of your shopping should be quite easy. See *Useful Addresses* at the back of the book for mail order suppliers.

There is one product that you may have difficulty in obtaining, and this is milk-free margarine. Almost all margarines and similar spreads contain whey and/or milk solids. However, to comply with strict dietary laws, Kosher margarines are milk-free and are available from shops which specialize in foods for the Jewish community. The most widely available brand in the UK is *Tomor*.

Once you have found a supply, buying in bulk and freezing it until needed is probably the easiest way of coping with your margarine problem. Fortunate people will be able to regularly buy a vegan margarine (which will be milk-free) at their local Health Store.

Some slimmer's low-fat spreads are milk-free but are not suitable for baking or cooking.

Special Baking Powder

Make your own baking powder (raising powder) and make sure that it does not contain wheat-flour or any milk by-product such as lactose.

Imperial (Metric)
¼ oz (7g) potassium bicarbonate
4¾ oz (115g) potato flour (farina)

American
2 teaspoonsful potassium
  bicarbonate
¾ cupful potato flour (farina)

Mix and store in a screwtop jar. Use as required. Potassium bicarbonate can be bought at chemists.

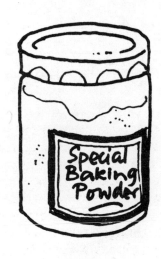

6.

THE KITCHEN FRONT

Many people imagine that a special diet means a lot of special and expensive gadgets as the food will be difficult to prepare. This is sheer nonsense. You will find only very basic items are needed in the way of kitchen tools. Here is a guide which will give you an idea of the tools needed.

1. *Kitchen knife.* This is probably the tool you will use most as you will need it to prepare vegetables and fruit — almost half the diet. It is important to buy one which feels comfortable and strong. An old-fashioned type with a wooden handle and a blade which is shaped to a point will serve you best. A small one and a slightly larger medium-sized one are all you need. If you buy good quality ones they will probably last you for 30 years!

2. *Chopping board.* With your knives you will need to use a chopping board. As most of the ones sold in the shops are too small, try a wooden pastry board.

3. *Soup ladle.* Soup is the most impossible food to handle without a ladle. If you try to pour it it will most likely splash everywhere and a tablespoon is just not large enough.

4. *Blender.* For making really smooth soups these are wonderful and need not cost a fortune.

5. *Sieve.* Use for straining soups and for straining small amounts of vegetables. Metal ones are preferable to plastic as they are heat-proof.

6. *Wooden spoons.* These are essential for stirring and are all you need for mixing cakes etc. An electric mixer is not essential.

7. *Saucepans.* A set of saucepans in varying sizes with tight-fitting lids is a must. A frying pan (skillet) with deep sides is useful for stir-frying vegetables if you don't want to go to the expense of buying a wok.

8. *Rolling pin.* A plain wooden one will give you good service and will be unbreakable.

9. *A selection of bowls and basins.* Chip-proof glass ones are probably the most hard-wearing.

10. *Baking sheets and trays.* Just ordinary ones will do. There is no need to get specially coated, non-stick kinds.

11. *Colanders.* Be careful when buying these. Some on the market are more for decoration than use! Make sure you get one with plenty of holes for draining. A small one is often useful for draining just a small amount of vegetables; a large one is useful for potatoes and rice.

12. *Grapefruit knife.* This really makes preparing a grapefruit easy. It should have a curved double edge which is serrated.

13. *Garlic press or crusher.* Ignore the pretty plastic ones. Buy a metal one which will be strong enough to press a clove of garlic.

14. *Kitchen scissors.* Good for cutting up parsley and herbs when you are in too much of a hurry to chop them.

15. *Oven gloves.* These are really much safer to use than a trailing tea-towel and do protect your hands all over from burns.

16. *Pastry cutters.* Again, avoid the pretty plastic ones which begin life completely blunt and stay that way! The old-fashioned metal ones are the best.

17. *Grater.* The easiest type to use is round with a handle at the top.

7.
EMERGENCY MENUS

As it will take a few days or perhaps even a few weeks, depending where you live, to get organized with a new eating regime, here are some suggestions for menus using readily available ingredients. This should enable you to begin the new diet immediately instead of waiting until you have bought all the special foods you might need.

Breakfasts
Savoury Breakfast Cakes (see page 36).

or Muesli with rice base (see page 38).

or 2 slices grilled back bacon, grilled tomatoes and fried potato (pre-cooked the day before).

Drinks: Pure fruit juice, black coffee or tea with lemon.

Mid-morning
Drinks: Black coffee or tea with lemon.

Few sultanas (golden seedless raisins) or raisins and shelled almonds.

Lunch
Fish canned in oil or water — sardines, tuna or salmon, plus baked jacket potato, large mixed salad of lettuce, cucumber, grated carrot, tomato, dressed with wine vinegar, oil, a sprinkle of raw cane sugar and sea salt and freshly ground black pepper.

Follow with an apple or pear.

Drink: Water.

Mid-afternoon
Drinks: Black coffee, lemon or herb tea.

1 banana or apple, or other fresh fruit in season.

Dinner
Fruit juice followed by grilled lamb or pork chop or grilled steak with lightly cooked green vegetables and plain boiled potatoes or rice. No gravy except the vegetable juices.

Alternatively: use the Beef Casserole with Orange recipe on page 84 or Good Old Fashioned Stew (see page 90).

End the meal with a fresh fruit salad.

If you feel hungry at any time during the day eat raisins and plain shelled nuts. If you are not used to black coffee or lemon tea, drink just plain water.

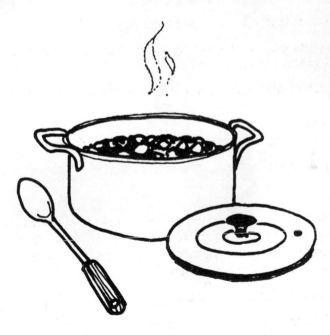

8.

BASICS

There are some foods or special items you will wish to eat or use every day and at any time of the day, perhaps even at every meal. Here are the basic recipes you will need for these:

Staples

Without wheat (or rye, barley and oats that have not been contaminated by wheat) making bread can be difficult. It is worth trying suitable types of crispbread to see if they can be tolerated. Look at the ingredients list of the packet or carton and check with the lists given in this book to see if they are wheat-free, milk-free and egg-free.

If available, *Trufree* flours are guaranteed wheat-free and are suitable as they do not contain lactose (a milk product) or egg. They can also be made into bread etc., without adding milk or egg. (Failing this, it is best to make your own flour blend at home from permitted ingredients and use as required. See Brown Bread Flour page 32.)

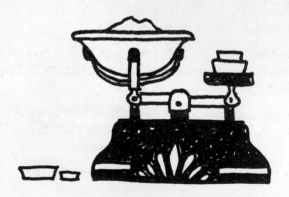

BREAD DOUGH FOR CRUSTY ROLLS AND BREADSTICKS

Imperial (Metric)	American
10 oz (275g) *Trufree* No. 4 flour	10 ounces *Trufree* No. 4 flour
¼ oz sachet (7g) special yeast provided	1 sachet special yeast provided
3 pinches sea salt	3 pinches of sea salt
1 heaped teaspoonful raw cane sugar	1 heaped teaspoonful raw cane sugar
1 oz (25g) milk-free margarine	2½ tablespoonsful milk-free margarine
5 fl oz (150ml) warm water	⅔ cupful warm water

1. Put the flour, yeast, salt and sugar into a bowl. Mix well.

2. Add the margarine and rub in with the fingers.

3. Pour in the warm water and mix to a sticky dough. Knead, without adding more flour, to one ball of dough. If you find it too stiff, add a little more warm water.

4. Take the ball of dough and knead on a cool worktop, again without adding more flour. After a couple of minutes the doughs should be smooth and shiny.

5. Shape and bake as directed for rolls and breadsticks.

CRUSTY ROLLS

1. Make the Bread Dough recipe as above.

2. For each roll use about 1 oz (25g) of dough. Roll into small sausage shapes or round, flattened rolls and place on an oiled baking sheet, leaving them to rise in a warm place.

3. When doubled in size (about 15 to 20 minutes, usually), bake on the top shelf of an oven preheated to 425°F/220°C (Gas Mark 7). Baking time is about 15 minutes.

4. Put on to a wire rack to cool and eat freshly baked.

BREADSTICKS

1. Make the Bread Dough recipe (page 31).

2. For each breadstick allow about ½ oz (15g) dough. Roll into long pencil shapes and place on an oiled baking sheet to rise in a warm place. This may only take a few minutes and the shapes will neaten themselves considerably as they rise.

3. Bake on the top shelf of a preheated oven 425°F/220°C (Gas Mark 7) for about 9 or 10 minutes, until golden and crusty. Cool on a wire rack and eat on the day they are baked.

BROWN BREAD FLOUR
Makes 4 loaves

Imperial (Metric)	American
4 oz (100g) soya flour	1 cupful soy flour
1 lb 2 oz (500g) ground brown rice	1 lb 2 oz ground brown rice
3 oz (75g) yellow split pea flour	6 tablespoonsful yellow split pea flour
2 tablespoonsful dried pectin	2 tablespoonsful dried pectin
2 oz (50g) ground almonds	4 tablespoonsful ground almonds
1 heaped tablespoonful carob powder	1 heaped tablespoonful carob powder

1. Put all ingredients, carefully weighed,* into a large mixing bowl. Mix well, by hand.

2. Put into a polythene bag, seal and use as required. Best stored in the fridge.

*Weights need to be accurate for best results and the imperial measures are the best ones to use.

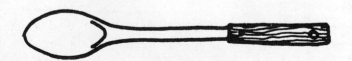

BROWN BREAD

Imperial (Metric)	American
2 heaped teaspoonsful dried yeast granules	2 heaped teaspoonsful dried yeast granules
9 fl oz (250ml) warm water	1¼ cupsful warm water
1 heaped teaspoonful raw cane sugar	1 heaped teaspoonful raw cane sugar
7¼ oz (210g) brown bread flour (see recipe page 32)	1¾ cupsful brown bread flour (see recipe page 32)
3 pinches sea salt	3 pinches sea salt
1 tablespoonful sunflower oil	1 tablespoonful sunflower oil

1. Preheat oven at 350°F/180°C (Gas Mark 4).

2. Sprinkle the yeast granules into the warm water. Add the sugar and stir.

3. Leave for a few minutes so that the yeast can soften.

4. Put the flour into a bowl with the sea salt and oil. Mix.

5. Stir the yeast and pour on to the flour.

6. Mix well to a smooth, creamy batter.

7. Grease a loaf tin size 7¼ × 3½ × 2¼ in (185 × 90 × 50mm) with oil and flour with ground rice or maize flour (cornstarch).

8. Spoon/pour into the prepared tin and put straight into the preheated oven on the top shelf.

9. Bake for about 1 hour, until well risen, brown and crusty.

10. Turn out onto a wire rack to cool as soon as you take it out of the oven. Do not cut until cold as the loaf needs to 'set'.

Note: Use as ordinary bread and store in a polythene bag, sealed. You can make this loaf with fresh yeast — use double the amount given. This loaf is not made or baked in the same way as ordinary bread. As the loaf does not contain gluten the yeast will not behave in the usual way. This is why it does not need to be left to rise and why it is cooked on such a low temperature.

CRISPBREADS

Imperial (Metric)	American
1 oz (25g) rice bran	2 tablespoonsful rice bran
3 pinches sea salt	3 pinches sea salt
7 oz (180g) *Trufree* No. 6 flour	1¾ cupsful *Trufree* No. 6 flour
2 oz (50g) milk-free margarine	4 tablespoonsful milk-free margarine
Approx. 6 tablespoonsful cold water	Approx. 6 tablespoonsful cold water

1. Preheat oven at 450°F/230°C (Gas Mark 8).

2. Mix the bran, salt and flour in a bowl.

3. Put in the margarine and rub in with the fingers.

4. Pour in the water and mix to one lump of dough. Don't worry if it is too sticky as the water releases the binder in the flour.

5. Use more flour to roll out thinly. (Do this in two batches if you find it easier.) Cut into rectangles or squares.

6. Lift them on to ungreased baking sheets with a spatula. Prick all over with a fork.

7. Bake for about 15 minutes on the top shelf.

8. Place on to a wire rack to cool and crisp.

9. Store in an air tight tin.

Note: Do not overbake these crispbreads. They should be a pale yellow colour and golden brown at the edges. Recrisp any which go soft by putting them on a baking sheet and baking them for 2 or 3 minutes in the oven.

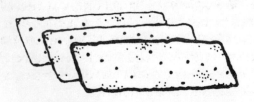

9.

BREAKFASTS

This is probably the greatest problem meal for a wheat-free, egg-free, milk-free dieter. With the traditional breakfast being egg based with wheat cereals and milk, other forms of protein must be used for this very important first meal of the day. As this section relies on simple dishes most come as suggestions and not recipes.

If sitting down to breakfast becomes a misery when you have to watch the rest of the family tucking in to all the things you are not allowed, take your breakfast on a tray, away from the table. Why not spoil yourself and have breakfast in bed?

If you like a large breakfast then fruit juice, fresh fruit or stewed fruit can be your starter. Follow with a protein dish such as grilled fish, baked beans or cold meat. If you are still hungry, try a non-wheat cereal moistened with soya milk. Tea or coffee without milk and you should be well set up for the morning! (You will undoubtedly be able to buy at least one kind of wheat-free breakfast cereal at your local health store or supermarket, and soya milk too, if you don't mind it.)

BUBBLE AND SQUEAK — to eat with cold meat or grilled bacon. This is a simple, traditional British dish. Chop left-over cooked greens and potato. Cook in a little sunflower oil to prevent it sticking. When brown on one side, turn over and brown on the other. Your finished dish should be a compressed flatish cake of vegetables, crisp and brown on the outside and soft in the middle.

SAVOURY BREAKFAST CAKES

Imperial (Metric)	American
2 oz (50g) cold, boiled potato	2 ounces cold, boiled potatoes
Generous knob of milk-free margarine	Generous knob of milk-free margarine
2 oz (50g) cold minced ham*	2 ounces cold minced ham*
Sprinkle of chopped parsley	Sprinkle of chopped parsley
Sea salt	Sea salt
Freshly gound black pepper	Freshly ground black pepper
Vegetable oil for frying	Vegetable oil for frying

1. Mash the potato with the margarine.

2. Put into a bowl and add the ham and parsley. Mix well.

3. Season to taste and shape into two round, flat cakes.

4. Heat a little oil in a frying pan.

5. Put in the savoury cakes and fry on both sides until browned.

6. Serve hot with grilled tomatoes, fried mushrooms and/or wheat-free baked beans in tomato sauce.

Note: Other kinds of meat can be used such as cold leftover beef or lamb from a joint. Bacon can be used too. Grill then chop into small pieces. Fish such as cold grilled haddock or cod (filleted) and canned salmon or tuna (in oil) will add variety. Drain off all the oil before flaking. If oatmeal can be eaten without ill-effects then the savoury cakes can be rolled in oatmeal before frying. This will give a crisper texture.

*Must be without breadcrumb coating.

BEANS ON FRIED BREAD

Fry slices of wheat-free bread in shallow hot oil until golden and crisp. Serve on a hot plate topped with wheat-free baked beans in tomato sauce, heated in a small saucepan. Grilled tomatoes, fried mushrooms and grilled bacon can be added to make the dish more substantial.

If the idea of fried bread does not appeal then try toasted wheat-free bread spread with milk-free margarine.

POTATO NEST

For this you will need a shallow fireproof dish that will fit under the grill. Put a generous portion of cold mashed potato (make sure it was mashed with milk-free margarine) into the dish and flatten with a knife. Put under a medium grill for about 10 minutes when the top will be crisp and the potato heated right through. Make a well in the centre through to the bottom of the dish. Fill this with hot, wheat-free baked beans in tomato sauce and top with a sprinkle of chopped grilled bacon or ham. Serve on a plate, still in the fireproof dish.

KEDGEREE

Mix 2 or 3 tablespoonsful cold, cooked brown rice with a chopped tomato, chopped ham, cold flaked dish, cooked peas or sweetcorn. Mix and season to taste. Heat a little oil in a frying pan and heat the mixture through. Serve on a hot plate. Freshly chopped parsley can also be added before serving.

WHITEBAIT — see section on Main Meals for this recipe. Makes a good protein-high breakfast.

GRILLED FISH — see section on Main Meals for this recipe. Serve with wheat-free bread and milk-free margarine.

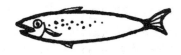

COLD MEAT WITH FRIED POTATO — choose from cold roast beef or lamb cut off a joint, or ham without breadcrumb coating. Fry cold, boiled potatoes left over from the day before, in a little sunflower oil and serve with grilled tomatoes or wheat-free and milk-free tomato sauce (see recipe, page 135).

MUESLI

For those people who cannot entertain the thought of a substantial breakfast a muesli might be the answer.

In a dish put 1 to 2 tablespoonsful of one of the suggested bases (see below). Sprinkle with 2 teaspoonsful of seeds. Add 1 piece of fresh fruit from the list and 1 heaped tablespoonful each of dried fruit and nuts. Sweeten with one of the suggested sweeteners and moisten with one of the liquids.

Bases: Cold cooked rice, *Trufree* Crispbran (if obtainable) rolled oats (if you can find a brand that you can tolerate without any ill-effects) or a non-wheat cereal.

Seeds: Sunflower seeds, sesame seeds.

Fresh fruit: Banana, apple, pear, nectarine, fresh plums, peach, strawberries, raspberries, sweet apricots and cherries, etc.

Dried fruit: Seedless raisins, sultanas (golden raisins), chopped dried apricots, peaches or stoned prunes.

Nuts: Any kind of plain nuts such as almonds, cashews, walnuts, hazelnuts, etc.

Sweetners: Liquid honey, fructose (fruit sugar) or raw cane sugar.

Liquid: Spring water, soya milk (if liked), fruit juice.

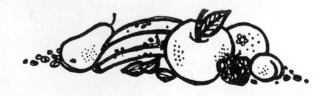

BREAKFAST PIZZA
(Serves 1)

Imperial (Metric)	American
1 oz (25g) milk-free margarine	1 heaped tablespoonful milk-free
2 oz (50g) ground brown rice	margarine
1½ oz (40g) finely grated apple	¼ cupful ground brown rice
Sunflower oil	¼ cupful finely grated apple
1 mushroom, sliced thinly	Sunflower oil
2 rashers back bacon, grilled	1 mushroom, sliced thinly
1 large tomato, sliced thinly	2 rashers back bacon, grilled
Sea salt	1 large tomato, sliced thinly
Freshly ground black pepper	Sea salt
	Freshly ground black pepper

1. Preheat oven at 425°F/220°C (Gas Mark 7).

2. Use a fork to blend the margarine, ground rice and apple. Knead into one ball of dough and press out by hand into a circle, on an oiled ovenproof plate. This will form the pizza base.

3. Brush with sunflower oil and arrange the mushroom slices over it.

4. Trim off all fat and rind from the bacon and discard. Chop bacon and sprinkle over the base.

5. Cover with a layer of tomato slices and season to taste.

6. Bake on the top of the oven for about 20 minutes.

7. Serve hot from the oven.

Optional: Sprinkle with ground nuts before baking, for extra protein.

Note: This also makes a good supper snack.

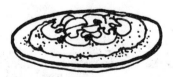

FRUIT PANCAKES

Imperial (Metric)	American
2 heaped tablespoonsful *Trufree* No. 6 or 7 flour	2 heaped tablespoonsful *Trufree* No. 6 or 7 flour
2 teaspoonsful vegetable oil	2 teaspoonsful vegetable oil
Water to mix	Water to mix
More vegetable oil for frying	More vegetable oil for frying
Sweetened stewed fruit (keep hot)	Sweetened stewed fruit (keep hot)

1. Mix the flour and oil in a basin.

2. Gradually add cold water, while you stir and beat until you have a thin, smooth batter.

3. Heat a little oil in a frying pan (skillet) until it begins to smoke. Pour in about 3 tablespoonsful of the batter and tilt the pan so that the batter covers the base of it.

4. Cook until crisp and browning, turning once with a spatula.

5. Spread each pancake with stewed fruit and stack one on top of the other. Serve right away.

Note: Any kind of fruit in season that will stew is suitable — apple, pear, plum, gooseberry, blackberry and apple, etc. Sweeten to taste.

With all these suggestions for breakfast, serve lemon tea or black coffee. For a good appetite also serve toasted special wheat-free bread, milk-free margarine and marmalade or honey.

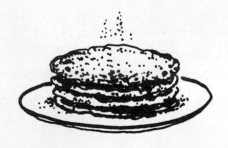

10.

SOUPS, STARTERS AND SNACKS

BROAD BEAN SOUP

This is a very creamy textured soup but made without cream or milk.

Imperial (Metric)	American
1 medium onion, peeled and sliced thinly	1 medium onion, peeled and sliced thinly
1 tablespoonful thin cooking oil	1 tablespoonful thin cooking oil
½ lb (225g) shelled broad beans	1½ cupsful shelled broad beans
1 tablespoonful thin, wheat-free soya sauce	1 tablespoonful thin, wheat-free soy sauce
1 pint (570ml) water	2½ cupsful water
Sea salt	Sea salt
Freshly ground black pepper	Freshly ground black pepper

1. Fry the onion in the oil until transparent but not brown.

2. Put in the broad beans, wheat-free soya sauce and about two thirds of the water.

3. Bring to the boil and simmer with the lid on for about 20 minutes for small young beans and up to 10 minutes longer for older ones. (Frozen ones will only need about 4 to 5 minutes).

4. Remove from heat and liquidize with the rest of the water.

5. Taste and season. If you find the taste a little 'metallic' this can be rectified with a few pinches of raw cane sugar.

6. Serve hot.

FRESH PEA SOUP

Imperial (Metric)
1 medium onion, peeled and sliced
2 teaspoonsful vegetable oil
¾ pint (400ml) water
¾ lb (350g) fresh peas, after
    shelling
2 teaspoonsful wheat-free soya
    sauce
Sea salt and freshly ground black
    pepper

American
1 medium onion, peeled and sliced
2 teaspoonsful vegetable oil
2 cupsful water
2 cupsful fresh peas, after shelling
2 teaspoonsful wheat-free soy sauce
Sea salt and freshly ground black
    pepper

1. Fry the onion in the oil until transparent.

2. Add half the water, the peas and the soya sauce. Bring to the boil and simmer with the lid on for about 8-10 minutes.

3. Pour in the rest of the water, and liquidize.

4. Return to saucepan, season to taste and serve hot.

LENTIL SOUP

Imperial (Metric)
5 oz (125g) lentils
2 medium onions, peeled and sliced
1 tablespoonful vegetable oil
1 medium potato, peeled and sliced
    thinly
1 tablespoonful wheat-free soya
    sauce
1 pint (½ litre) water
Sea salt and freshly ground black
    pepper

American
¾ cupful lentils
2 medium onions, peeled and sliced
1 tablespoonful vegetable oil
1 medium potato, peeled and sliced
    thinly
1 tablespoonful wheat-free soy
    sauce
2½ cupsful water
Sea salt and freshly ground black
    pepper

1. Wash the lentils in a wire sieve and soak overnight in a large bowl with 1 pint plus (550ml plus) of water.

2. Fry the onion in the oil, using a large pan.

3. Add the potato, soya sauce, the strained lentils, the water and seasoning.

4. Bring to the boil and simmer for 40 minutes.

5. Remove from heat and allow to cool. Liquidize.

6. Serve hot with special bread sippets.

AVOCADO SOUP
(Serves 2)

This is an unusual soup that must be served as soon as it is made or it will discolour. Like Broad Bean Soup the final result is very creamy without adding milk or cream.

Imperial (Metric)	American
1 small onion, peeled and sliced finely	1 small onion, peeled and sliced finely
1 teaspoonful milk-free margarine	1 teaspoonful milk-free margarine
1 medium avocado pear	1 medium avocado pear
2 teaspoonsful wheat-free (thin) soya sauce	2 teaspoonsful wheat-free (thin) soy sauce
½ pint (¼ litre) water	2½ cupsful water
Sea salt	Sea salt
Freshly ground black pepper	Freshly ground black pepper

1. Fry the onion in the margarine until transparent but not brown.

2. Peel the avocado and remove the stone.

3. Put fried onion and avocado (cut into pieces) into the blender with the wheat-free soya sauce and water. Liquidize.

4. Return to saucepan, heat and simmer for 3 or 4 minutes.

5. Season to taste and serve right away.

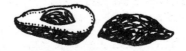

CAULIFLOWER SOUP

Make and serve immediately. A very creamy soup with a subtle flavour.

Imperial (Metric)	American
1 small onion, peeled and sliced finely	1 small onion, peeled and sliced finely
1 teaspoonful milk-free margarine	1 teaspoonful milk-free margarine
½ small cauliflower head	½ small cauliflower head
½ pint (285ml) water	2½ cupsful water
1 teaspoonful maize flour	1 teaspoonful cornstarch
Pinch grated nutmeg	Pinch grated nutmeg
1 teaspoonful wheat-free soya sauce	1 teaspoonful wheat-free soy sauce
Sea salt and freshly ground black pepper	Sea salt and freshly ground black pepper

1. Fry the onion in the margarine until transparent.

2. Cut the cauliflower into small pieces and put into the saucepan with half the water.

3. Bring to the boil and simmer for 5 minutes to soften. Remove from heat.

4. Mix the maize (cornstarch) with the remaining water and pour into the liquidizer goblet with the mixture from the saucepan.

5. Add the nutmeg and soya sauce.

6. Heat through and simmer for another 4 or 5 minutes while you stir.

7. Taste, season and serve hot, immediately.

Note: The cauliflower should have creamy white curds and be nice and crisp. Avoid discoloured rubbery ones as they will be far from fresh.

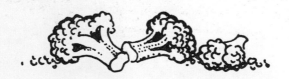

FRENCH COUNTRY SOUP

Imperial (Metric)
1 lb (½ kilo) leeks, trimmed
3 carrots, trimmed
1½ tablespoonsful vegetable oil
1 lb (½ kilo) potatoes, peeled
1½ pints (¾ litre) water
1 tablespoonful wheat-free soya
  sauce
Sea salt and freshly ground black
  pepper
1 heaped tablespoonful finely
  chopped fresh parsley

American
1 pound leeks, trimmed
3 carrots, trimmed
1½ tablespoonsful vegetable oil
1 pound potatoes, peeled
3¾ cupsful water
1 tablespoonful wheat-free soy
  sauce
Sea salt and freshly ground black
  pepper
1 heaped tablespoonful finely
  chopped fresh parsley

1. Cut the leeks in half lengthways. Wash well and cut into small sections.

2. Chop the carrots into small pieces and fry in the oil with the leeks, while stirring, for about 5 minutes.

3. Add the potato, cut into thin slices and about two-thirds of the water. Also add the soya sauce, then bring to the boil and simmer with the lid on for about 20 to 25 minutes.

4. Remove from heat and add the rest of the water. Liquidize in a blender and return to saucepan. Taste and season.

5. Reheat and stir in the chopped parsley. Serve hot.

Note: The potatoes make this a very filling soup. Serve to the whole family.

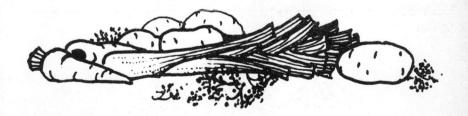

VEGETABLE CASSEROLE
(Serves 1)

Imperial (Metric)	American
3 medium mushrooms	3 medium mushrooms
1 medium tomato	1 medium tomato
2 thin slices onion	2 thin slices onion
1 small stick celery	1 small stalk celery
1 teaspoonful wheat-free soya sauce	1 teaspoonful wheat-free soy sauce
1 teaspoonful white wine or white wine vinegar	1 teaspoonful white wine or white wine vinegar
2 tablespoonsful water	2 tablespoonsful water
1 teaspoonful freshly chopped parsley	1 teaspoonful freshly chopped parsley
Sea salt	Sea salt
Freshly ground black pepper	Freshly ground black pepper

1. Preheat oven 350°F/180°C (Gas Mark 4).

2. Slice the mushrooms and tomatoes. Separate the onion into rings and chop the celery finely.

3. In a small casserole, pack the vegetables in layers, ending with a layer of mushrooms. Press down well.

4. In a cup mix the soya sauce, wine or vinegar and water. Pour over the vegetables. Lastly sprinkle with the chopped parsley. Season to taste.

5. Put on the lid and bake for about 30 minutes until the vegetables are tender. Serve hot or cold.

Note: Make sure you press the vegetables down well before cooking or the top layer will be dry.

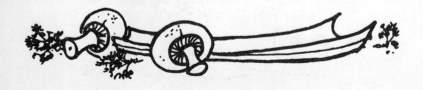

ONION AND POTATO SOUP

Imperial (Metric)
1 large onion, peeled and sliced
   thinly
1 tablespoonful sunflower oil
1 clove garlic, peeled and chopped
2 medium potatoes, peeled and
   sliced
¾ pint (400ml) cold water
2 teaspoonsful wheat-free soya
   sauce
Sea salt and freshly ground black
   pepper

American
1 large onion, peeled and sliced
   thinly
1 tablespoonful sunflower oil
1 clove garlic, peeled and chopped
2 medium potatoes, peeled and
   sliced
2 cupsful cold water
2 teaspoonsful wheat-free soy sauce
Sea salt and freshly ground black
   pepper

1. Fry the onion in the oil for 3 or 4 minutes.

2. Crush in the garlic and stir.

3. Add the potato, half the water and the soya sauce. Heat through and simmer for about 10 to 12 minutes with the lid on.

4. Remove from heat, add the remaining water and liquidize in a blender.

5. Pour back into the saucepan and season to taste.

6. Serve hot.

Optional: Sprinkle in a little freshly chopped parsley, just before serving.

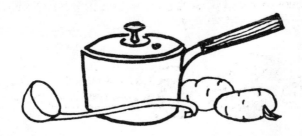

MUSHROOM AND TOMATO SOUP

Imperial (Metric)
1 medium onion, peeled and sliced
1 tablespoonful vegetable oil
4 oz (100g) fresh mushrooms,
   washed and sliced
¾ pint (400ml) tomato juice
2 teaspoonsful wheat-free soya
   sauce
Sea salt and freshly ground black
   pepper

American
1 medium onion, peeled and sliced
1 tablespoonful vegetable oil
2 cupsful fresh mushrooms, washed
   and sliced
2 cupsful tomato juice
2 teaspoonsful wheat-free soy sauce
Sea salt and freshly ground black
   pepper

1. Fry the onion in the oil for 3 to 4 minutes.

2. Put the fried onion, mushroom slices, water and soya sauce into a liquidizer, blend and pour into the saucepan.

3. Bring to the boil and simmer for about 5 minutes.

4. Season to taste and serve hot.

SIPPETS

Fry cubes of special wheat-free bread lightly in hot vegetable oil until golden. Sprinkle into hot soup and serve. Cut the bread into thick slices and then into cubes, before you fry them.

MUSHROOMS WITH MINT
(Serves 1)

Imperial (Metric)
1 tablespoonful sunflower oil
½ clove garlic, peeled
4 oz (100g) mushrooms
2 fresh tomatoes, peeled and
   chopped
Fresh mint leaves, chopped
Sea salt
Freshly ground black pepper

American
1 tablespoonful sunflower oil
½ clove garlic, peeled
1 cupful mushrooms
2 fresh tomatoes, peeled and
   chopped
Fresh mint leaves, chopped
Sea salt
Freshly ground black pepper

1. Heat the oil in a frying pan (skillet).

2. Put in the garlic (crushed), mushrooms, tomatoes and chopped mint.

3. Season and cover with a lid.

4. Simmer for about 12 to 15 minutes.

5. Serve hot with triangles of wheat-free fried bread or sippets.

WHITEBAIT

Imperial (Metric)	American
4 oz (100g) whitebait	4 ounces whitebait
Maize flour	Cornmeal
3 tablespoonsful sunflower or soya oil	3 tablespoonsful sunflower or soy oil
Sea salt and freshly ground black pepper	Sea salt and freshly ground black pepper
Parsley sprigs	Parsley sprigs
Lemon slice for decoration	Lemon slice for decoration

1. Wash the fish well under the cold running tap. Drain well in a colander.

2. Put a tablespoonful of maize flour (cornmeal) into a paper bag and toss the fish in this until well coated.

4. Heat the oil in a shallow pan and fry the coated fish in this a few at a time. When crisp and brown, drain on kitchen paper and keep hot while you fry the remainder.

5. Serve right away with the parsley and lemon garnish.

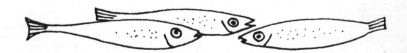

TOMATO STARTER
(Serves 1)

A very simple but delicious starter. Use a really good quality tomato — a home grown one would be ideal.

Imperial (Metric)	American
1 tomato	1 tomato
1 level teaspoonful freshly chopped parsley	1 level teaspoonful freshly chopped parsley
1 slice onion, chopped very finely	1 slice onion, chopped very finely
Raw cane sugar	Raw cane sugar
Freshly ground black pepper	Freshly ground black pepper
Sea salt	Sea salt

1. Cut the tomato into thin slices.

2. Lay overlapping, on a plate, and sprinkle with the parsley and onion plus a few pinches of sugar.

3. Season to taste.

4. Serve cold with wheat-free crispbread and milk-free margarine.

LIVER AND MUSHROOM PÂTÉ

Imperial (Metric)	American
½ lb (¼ kilo) chicken livers	8 ounces chicken livers
½ medium onion, peeled and chopped	½ medium onion, peeled and chopped
1 tablespoonful sunflower oil	1 tablespoonful sunflower oil
1 clove garlic, peeled	1 clove garlic, peeled
½ lb (¼ kilo) mushrooms, chopped	8 ounces mushrooms, chopped
¼ teaspoonful dried thyme	¼ teaspoonful dried thyme
Sea salt	Sea salt
Freshly ground black pepper	Freshly ground black pepper

1. Cut out all the strings etc., from the livers and discard.

2. Wash and chop livers. Pat dry with kitchen paper.

3. Fry the onion in the oil until soft.

4. Add the chopped livers and crush in the garlic. Turn up the heat and stir with a small wooden spoon or fork. As soon as the livers start to turn brown and crumble, add the mushrooms.

5. Cook while you stir for about 3 or 4 minutes.

6. Leave to cool, then blend, adding the thyme and seasoning to taste.

7. Put into little dishes and store, covered, in the fridge.

Note: Serve with hot wheat-free toast and milk-free margarine for the special dieter and ordinary bread and butter for the rest of the family. A useful starter as it will serve the whole family and can be made well in advance.

CRUDITÉS

Serve as dips with special mayonnaise as a starter.

Radishes — scrubbed and trimmed.

Celery — scrubbed and trimmed and cut into short lengths.

Carrot — washed and trimmed and cut into matchstick shapes.

Spring onions (scallions) — washed and trimmed.

Cauliflower — use the crisp white pieces and break into florets after washing well.

Lettuce — use just the heart leaves. Wash and pat dry with a clean tea-towel. Any variety of lettuce will do.

Tomato — only use if you can get small fruits. Wash and leave whole.

Cucumber — leave the skin on and cut into small fingers.

Sprouting Broccoli — use just the small florets after washing.

STUFFED MUSHROOMS
(Serves 1)

Although this makes an unusual starter it can also be a good accompaniment to baked fish or chicken.

Imperial (Metric)	American
3 open, largish mushrooms	3 open, largish mushrooms
1 tablespoonful sunflower oil	1 tablespoonful sunflower oil
½ small onion, peeled and chopped finely	½ small onion, peeled and chopped finely
1 tablespoonful wheat-free breadcrumbs	1 tablespoonful wheat-free breadcrumbs
1 rasher back bacon, grilled	1 rasher back bacon, grilled
2 heaped teaspoonsful chopped fresh parsley	2 heaped teaspoonsful chopped fresh parsley
1 heaped teaspoonful ground almonds	1 heaped teaspoonful ground almonds
Garlic salt	Garlic salt
Freshly ground black pepper	Freshly ground black pepper
Parsley for garnish	Parsley for garnish

1. Preheat oven 375°F/190°C (Gas Mark 5).

2. Wash the mushrooms and remove stalks. Chop just the stalks finely.

3. Heat the oil in a frying pan (skillet) and put in the chopped stalks and onion. Fry over a gentle heat for about 3 to 4 minutes.

4. Sprinkle in the breadcrumbs and fry until brown and crisp.

5. Trim the fat off the grilled bacon and discard. Chop the bacon and add to the fried mixture with the chopped parsley and ground almonds.

6. Season with the garlic salt and pepper to taste.

7. Put the mushroom caps, hollow side up, in a well oiled, shallow, ovenproof dish. Fill the caps with stuffing.

8. Sprinkle with a little oil, cover with a lid and bake for about 25 minutes above centre of oven.

9. Serve hot, garnished with parsley.

Note: If preferred lean ham can be used instead of bacon. Just chop and add to stuffing mixture. If you don't have any wheat-free bread to spare try chopped, cold, boiled potato instead.

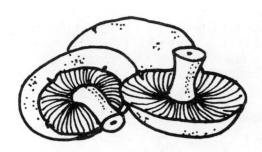

SUGGESTIONS FOR OTHER STARTERS
Other, old favourites that can be served to all the family are melon sprinkled with a little raw cane sugar (if not sweet enough), or a mixture of grapefruit and orange slices, or just plain grapefruit.

SNACKS

As most commercial biscuits are made with wheat-flour, egg and margarine (which is not milk-free), you will need to make your own biscuits at home if you wish to continue eating them for snacks. Here is a selection of special biscuit recipes to fill this gap. Store the end results in air-tight containers.

GINGER THINS

Imperial (Metric)
1 oz (25g) milk-free margarine
2 tablespoonsful black treacle
1 oz (25g) raw cane sugar
3 oz (75g) *Trufree* No. 7 S.R. flour
1/2 teaspoonful ground ginger

American
2 1/2 tablespoonsful milk-free
  margarine
2 tablespoonsful molasses
1 1/2 tablespoonsful raw cane sugar
1/3 cupful *Trufree* No. 7 S.R. flour
1/2 teaspoonful ground ginger

1. Preheat oven at 375°F/190°C (Gas Mark 5).

2. Melt the first three ingredients in a saucepan. Cool for 2 minutes.

3. Sift in the flour and ginger and mix well.

4. Liberally grease* baking sheets. Put teaspoonsful of the mixture on to the baking sheets leaving plenty of space around each one as they will spread a good deal during baking.

5. Flatten slightly with a knife and bake above centre of oven until brown.

6. Leave on the baking sheets to cool for a minute and then loosen and lift off carefully with a spatula.

7. Cool on a wire rack. As they cool down they will go crisp. Do not overbake or they will be too crumbly.

Variation: Use cinnamon instead of ginger for Cinnamon Thins.

*Use a milk-free margarine for greasing.

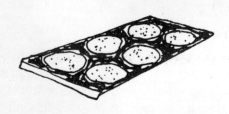

DIGESTIVE BISCUITS

Imperial (Metric)
1½ oz (40g) yellow split pea flour
1 oz (25g) ground brown rice
1 oz (25g) raw cane sugar
½ oz (15g) soya flour
3 pinches of powdered cloves
1 oz (25g) special milk-free
  margarine
A little water
Extra ground brown rice for rolling
  out

American
¼ cupful yellow split pea flour
2½ tablespoonsful ground brown
  rice
2½ tablespoonsful raw cane sugar
1 tablespoonful soy flour
3 pinches of powdered cloves
2½ tablespoonsful special milk-free
  margarine
A little water
Extra ground brown rice for rolling
  out

1. Preheat oven at 325°F/170°C (Gas Mark 3).

2. Put the first five ingredients into a bowl and mix well.

3. Add the margarine and rub in until the mixture resembles breadcrumbs.

4. Add water, 1 teaspoonful at a time, kneading the mixture until it binds. It should form one ball of dough and leave the bowl clean.

5. Roll out using more ground rice to about ⅛ in. (3mm) thick.

6. Cut into rounds with a pastry cutter and use a spatula to lift them on to a baking sheet.

7. Prick with a fork and bake for about 10 to 12 minutes.

8. Lift off carefully while still warm and leave to cool on a wire rack, when they will go crisp.

9. Store in an air-tight tin.

Note: This recipe should yield about a dozen biscuits.

SPICED FRUIT COOKIES

Imperial (Metric)	American
2 oz (50g) milk-free margarine	¼ cupful milk-free margarine
4 oz (100g) ground brown rice	½ cupful ground brown rice
3 oz (75g) finely grated eating apple	1 small eating apple, finely grated
1½ oz (40g) raw cane sugar	2 tablespoonsful raw cane sugar
1½ oz (40g) dried fruit — currants, sultanas, raisins, etc.	¼ cupful dried fruit — currants, golden seedless raisins, raisins, etc.
½ teaspoonful mixed spice	½ teaspoonful mixed spice

1. Preheat oven at 450°F/230°C (Gas Mark 8).

2. Put the margarine and ground rice into a bowl and blend with a fork.

3. Add the remaining ingredients and mix with a wooden spoon until it forms one ball of dough.

4. Oil a baking sheet and drop 10 spoonsful of the mixture on to it.

5. Spread out with a knife into cookie shapes about ¼ in. (6mm) thick.

6. Bake above centre of oven for 20 to 25 minutes. Allow to cool for a minute and then remove carefully with a spatula and put on to a wire rack to cool.

7. The cookies will crisp as they cool down. When cold, sprinkle with a little more sugar. Eat on the day of baking.

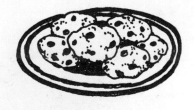

FRUIT AND NUTS

A simple snack and one that is easy to carry, combining fruit and nuts. Fruit can be fresh or dried but nuts should be fresh and not processed in any way. Wash dried fruits under the tap and dry on a clean tea-towel.

Try some of these combinations:

a. Dried apricots, raisins and almonds.

b. Sultanas (golden seedless raisins), cashews and a fresh banana.

c. Apple, raisins and hazelnuts/almonds.

d. Dried peaches, almonds and raisins.

e. Fresh pear with almonds and cashews.

f. Raisins, sultanas (golden seedless raisins), peanuts, almonds and hazelnuts.

After preparing, put into a small container with a lid or a small plastic bag. These are very high in calories, so if weight loss is a worry, this type of snack could prove very useful.

You will find most health stores carry a good selection of dried fruits and nuts. Once you have bought a selection you can make up little snacks and store them in small plastic bags in a container so that you may take one out when you want it. This should replace the biscuit tin in your life!

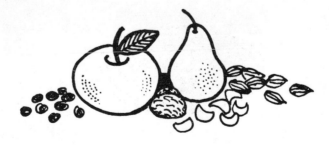

11.

MAIN MEALS

Without wheat, milk and eggs you will not be able to offer omelettes, quiches, pastas, sauces made with milk or anything which contains cheese. Dishes where eggs are used as a binder and where wheat is used for coating are also not on the menu. This means no rissoles, croquettes, fish in batter or breadcrumbs. The main source of carbohydrate will be brown rice and potatoes. Traditional roast lamb or beef (a joint) is permitted but not Yorkshire pudding to go with the beef. Although at first glance it seems as if main meals will have to be rather plain, you will find in this section recipes based on Italian, Indian, French and Chinese food as well as British, adapted for this rather special diet. This should make main mealtimes much more exciting than for an ordinary diet.

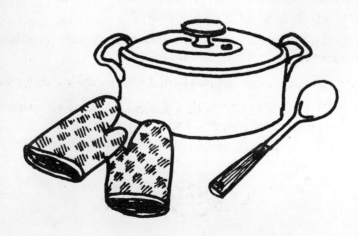

PRAWNS ITALIAN

Imperial (Metric)
1 medium onion, peeled and
  chopped finely
1 tablespoonful sunflower oil or
  similar
2 cloves garlic, peeled
2 oz (50g) mushrooms, sliced
½ medium green pepper, de-seeded
  and sliced thinly
4 medium tomatoes, peeled and
  chopped
3 teaspoonsful wheat-free soya
  sauce
½ lb (¼ kilo) peeled prawns
Sea salt and freshly ground black
  pepper
2 tablespoonsful finely chopped fresh
  parsley

American
1 medium onion, peeled and
  chopped finely
1 tablespoonful sunflower oil or
  similar
2 cloves garlic, peeled
1 cupful mushrooms, sliced
½ medium green pepper, de-seeded
  and sliced thinly
4 medium tomatoes, peeled and
  chopped
3 teaspoonsful wheat-free soy sauce
8 ounces peeled prawns
Sea salt and freshly ground black
  pepper
2½ tablespoonsful finely chopped
  fresh parsley

1. Fry the onion in the oil.

2. Crush in the garlic, using a garlic press.

3. Add the mushrooms, green pepper and tomatoes. Bring to the boil and simmer gently for 5 minutes.

4. Add the soya sauce and prawns. Heat through gently and simmer for another 5 minutes. Season to taste.

5. Serve hot, on a bed of plain boiled rice, sprinkled with parsley.

Note: This can be served with a green side salad of lettuce and cucumber, dressed with an oil and vinegar dressing.

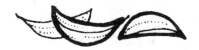

SHEPHERD'S PIE
(3 servings)

Imperial (Metric)	American
1 medium onion, peeled and chopped	1 medium onion, peeled and chopped
1 small clove of garlic, peeled	1 small clove of garlic, peeled
1 tablespoonful sunflower oil	1 tablespoonful sunflower oil
1 tomato, chopped	1 tomato, chopped
¾ lb minced lamb from precooked joint trimmed of fat etc. before cooking	3 cupsful minced lamb from precooked joint trimmed of fat etc. before cooking
1 medium carrot, grated coarsely	1 medium carrot, grated coarsely
3 teaspoonsful wheat-free soya sauce	3 teaspoonsful wheat-free soy sauce
3 heaped teaspoonsful maize flour	3 heaped teaspoonsful cornstarch
¼ pint (150ml) water	⅔ cupful water
1 heaped teaspoonful freshly chopped parsley	1 heaped teaspoonful freshly chopped parsley
3 pinches dried thyme	3 pinches dried thyme
1 heaped teaspoonful tomato *purée*	1 heaped teaspoonful tomato paste
3 portions mashed potato*	3 portions mashed potato*
Sea salt and freshly ground black pepper	Sea salt and freshly ground black pepper

1. Use a saucepan to fry the onion and crushed garlic in the sunflower oil.

2. Add the tomato when the onion begins to brown. Stir while you cook until you have a brown sauce.

3. Put in the minced lamb and grated carrot. Fry gently for about 5 minutes while turning over with a wooden spoon or spatula.

4. Spoon in the wheat-free soya sauce.

5. Blend the maize flour and water in a cup. Mix well and add to pan.

6. Sprinkle in the parsley, thyme and tomato *purée*. Stir well and cook while stirring for another 10 minutes. Season to taste, adding

more water if it looks too dry.

7. Transfer to a hot pie dish and cover with the mashed potato. Texture with a fork and make a hole in the centre, right through to the meat, to let out the steam during cooking.

8. Bake in a preheated oven 375°F/190°C (Gas Mark 5) on the top shelf for about 20 minutes.

9. Serve hot, golden topped and crisp, with a selection of vegetables (hot).

* The mashed potato should be made with plain boiled potatoes, milk-free margarine and a little water.

Note: A tasty way to use up a joint of lamb that won't cut into any more slices. Fresh raw minced lamb can also be used for this recipe but the cooking time for stage 3 will need to be 10 minutes and for stage 6 about 30 to 40 minutes.

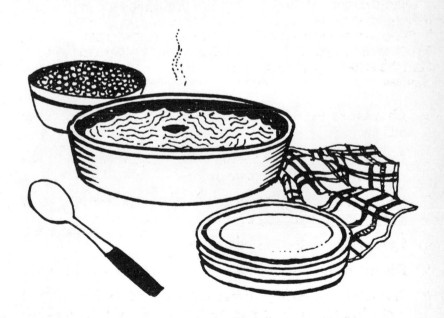

GOULASH
(Serves 4)

Imperial (Metric)	American
Maize flour	Cornstarch
Braising beef for 4 portions	Braising beef for 4 portions
3 medium onions, peeled	3 medium onions, peeled
Sunflower oil	Sunflower oil
1 medium tin tomatoes	1 medium can tomatoes
2 level teaspoonsful paprika	2 level teaspoonsful paprika
Sea salt	Sea salt

1. Sprinkle a little maize flour (cornstarch) on to a plate.

2. Trim off fat and gristle from meat and discard. Cut trimmed meat into neat cubes.

3. Roll in the maize flour (cornstarch).

4. Cut the onions into quarters and fry in a tablespoonful of oil, using a flameproof casserole.

5. Remove onions while you fry the beef cubes in another tablespoonful of the oil. Turn them over while you fry, to seal the meat.

6. Return onions to the casserole with the meat.

7. Add the tomatoes, paprika and seasoning. Bring to the boil, put on lid and transfer to a preheated oven 300°F/150°C (Gas Mark 2) about 2½ hours.

8. Serve with plain boiled rice and a green side salad. Garnish with fried wheat-free bread cut into triangles.

Note: This is a slow cooked casserole. Fresh tomatoes can be used instead of tinned but they will require peeling. If you find the gravy not rich enough then 2 or 3 teaspoonsful of wheat-free soya sauce can be added. A good deal of the success of this recipe depends on how tasty the tomatoes are. Some people will appreciate a little less paprika.

FISH AND CHIPS

1 portion cod, plaice or haddock, filleted and washed
Maize flour (cornmeal)
Sunflower or soya oil
1 portion peeled raw potatoes
Deep sunflower or soya oil for frying

Fish:

1. Dip the fish in maize flour (cornmeal) to coat it all over.

2. Heat a little oil in a frying pan (skillet).

3. Fry the fish for about 5 minutes on each side (or less if the fillet is thin) until cooked on the inside and with a crisp golden outside.

4. Drain on kitchen paper and serve hot.

Chips:

1. Cut the potato into 'fingers'.

2. Heat the oil until it begins to smoke slightly.

3. Put in the chips carefully, a few at a time so as not to make the fat bubble too much. Turn down the heat a little and cook for about 8 to 10 minutes or until the chips are golden and cooked through.

4. Drain on kitchen paper and serve immediately while piping hot.

Note: Don't fill the fat pan more than half full, as this is dangerous.

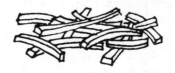

COLD SALMON
(Serves 2)

Imperial (Metric)	American
2 pints (1 litre) water	2 pints (1 litre) water
¼ pint (150ml) wine vinegar	¼ pint (150ml) wine vinegar
1 sliced onion	1 sliced onion
1 stick celery, chopped	1 stalk celery, chopped
1 carrot, grated coarsely	1 carrot, grated coarsely
1 heaped tablespoonful freshly chopped parsley	1 heaped tablespoonful freshly chopped parsley
1 teaspoonful black peppercorns	1 teaspoonful black peppercorns
Sea salt to taste	Sea salt to taste
2 fresh salmon steaks, washed, (cut from the centre of the fish)	2 fresh salmon steaks, washed, (cut from the centre of the fish)

1. Put the first seven ingredients into a large saucepan. Boil for about 30 minutes, adding more water if the level goes down too much.

2. Strain and pour back into the pan.

3. Add salt to taste and stir.

4. Put the salmon steaks carefully into the warm stock which should cover the fish. (If it doesn't, add more water.)

5. Bring to the boil and simmer for about 3 minutes.

6. Very carefully, using a large fish slice, turn the steaks over without breaking them.

7. Simmer for another 3 minutes and then turn out the heat.

8. Leave the salmon to grow cold in the liquid. It will continue to cook very slowly as it cools down.

9. Lift the fish out very carefully with a fish slice. Drain and put on to plates. Serve cold with salads and boiled new potatoes,

sprinkled with freshly chopped parsley and glazed with melted milk-free margarine.

Note: By leaving the salmon in the liquid until required for serving, it will not go dry. Serve for a special occasion — this is still considered to be a luxury fish.

TROUT

Trout can often be brought more cheaply than cod or haddock. The flesh is pale pink and has a delicate flavour. Buy trout already cleaned. Before cooking, wash and pat dry with kitchen paper. Season before all methods of cooking with sea salt and freshly ground black pepper.

Bake in an oiled, shallow, ovenproof dish that has a lid or cover. Preheat oven at 350°F/180°C (Gas Mark 4) for about 30 minutes, above centre of oven.

Fry on both sides for 5 or 6 minutes each side.

Grill on both sides for 8 to 10 minutes, under a medium grill. Traditional garnish for trout — lemon slices and sprigs of parsley.

Trout with Almonds

Fry the fish and wipe the pan clean. Fry a sprinkle of flaked almonds in a knob of milk-free margarine. Squeeze fresh lemon juice over the fish and cover with the fried almonds.

Baked Trout

Put the fish into a well-oiled dish and sprinkle with dried tarragon and 1 to 2 tablespoonsful white wine. Bake and serve with the juices.

Trout with Herbs

Coat the fish with maize flour (cornstarch) and fry. Keep hot while you heat a generous knob of milk-free margarine in a small pan. Squeeze in the juice of ¼ of a lemon and ½ level teaspoonful of mixed herbs. Mix well, pour over the fish and serve.

TROUT WITH MUSHROOMS
(Serves 1)

Imperial (Metric)	American
Sea salt	Sea salt
Freshly ground black pepper	Freshly ground black pepper
1 tablespoonful maize flour for coating	1 tablespoonful cornstarch for coating
1 trout, cleaned	1 trout, cleaned
Sunflower oil	Sunflower oil
2 spring onions (green part only)	2 scallions (green part only)
2 mushrooms, chopped	2 mushrooms, chopped
2 teaspoonsful lemon juice	2 teaspoonsful lemon juice
1 heaped teaspoonful chopped parsley	1 heaped teaspoonful chopped parsley
Parsley sprigs and lemon wedges	Parsley sprigs and lemon wedges

1. Sprinkle a little seasoning into the maize and coat the trout with this.

2. Put a little oil into a frying pan (skillet) and heat. Carefully put in the trout and fry on both sides for about 5 or 6 minutes, depending on the size of the fish. Keep hot.

3. In a separate pan heat about 2 teaspoonsful of the oil. Chop and fry the spring onion greens and the mushrooms — about 3 or 4 minutes will be enough.

4. Sprinkle the fish with the lemon juice and chopped parsley.

5. Put the cooked trout on to a hot plate and garnish with the onion/mushroom mixture. Decorate with parsley sprigs and lemon wedges.

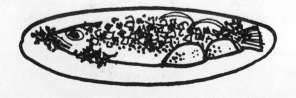

GRILLED WHITE FISH WITH HERBS
(Serves 1)

Imperial (Metric)
1 fillet of white fish*
Fresh lemon juice
1 tablespoonful freshly chopped
  parsley
1 tablespoonful freshly chopped
  chives
1 teaspoonful sunflower oil
Sea salt
Freshly ground black pepper

American
1 fillet of white fish*
Fresh lemon juice
1 tablespoonful freshly chopped
  parsley
1 tablespoonsful freshly chopped
  chives
1 teaspoonful sunflower oil
Sea salt
Freshly ground black pepper

1. Wash the fish of your choice.

2. Place on a metal plate or dish and sprinkle with the lemon juice, herbs, oil and seasoning.

3. Leave to marinate in the fridge for about half an hour.

4. Grill for about 4 to 5 minutes each side, under a moderate grill. If the fish starts to look dry sprinkle with a little more oil.

5. Serve hot with tomatoes (for colour), peas and plain boiled potatoes or rice. Also good with savoury rice.

Note: This recipe can be used for a breakfast dish if the chives are omitted. Serve hot with grilled tomatoes and wheat-free bread spread with milk-free margarine.

* Haddock, plaice, cod or turbot.

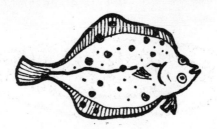

COD PORTUGAISE
(Serves 2)

Marinade:

Imperial (Metric)	American
3 tablespoonsful fresh lemon juice	3 tablespoonsful fresh lemon juice
3 tablespoonsful sunflower oil	3 tablespoonsful sunflower oil
Sea salt	Sea salt
Freshly ground black pepper	Freshly ground black pepper
1 clove garlic, peeled	1 clove garlic, peeled
1 bayleaf	1 bayleaf
4 cod fillets or steaks	4 cod fillets or steaks
Red sauce (page 69)	Red sauce (page 69)
Chopped parsley	Chopped parsley

1. Make the marinade by mixing the first six ingredients in a dish.

2. Put in the washed raw fish and leave for about 20 minutes. Turn the fish over and leave for another 20 minutes.

3. Preheat oven at 350°F/180°C (Gas Mark 4).

4. Grease an ovenproof dish with milk-free margarine or sunflower oil. Place the drained fish on this and put on the lid.

5. Bake for about 20 to 30 minutes, depending on thickness of fish.

6. Heat the Red sauce and pour a couple of tablespoonsful over each steak/fillet. Put back in the oven for five minutes.

7. Sprinkle with chopped parsley and serve hot with plain, boiled rice or potatoes and peas.

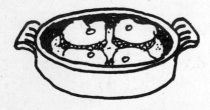

RED SAUCE
For fish, steak, chops, etc.

Imperial (Metric)
2 tablespoonsful sunflower oil
1 clove garlic, peeled
1 medium tin tomatoes
1 heaped teaspoonful tomato *purée*
Few pinches dried oregano
6 sprigs fresh parsley, chopped
  finely
1 teaspoonful raw cane sugar
Freshly ground black pepper
Sea salt

American
2 tablespoonsful sunflower oil
1 clove garlic, peeled
1 medium can tomatoes
1 heaped teaspoonful tomato paste
Few pinches dried oregano
6 sprigs fresh parsley, chopped
  finely
1 teaspoonful raw cane sugar
Freshly ground black pepper
Sea salt

1. Heat the oil in a small pan.

2. Crush in the garlic and lower the heat.

3. Chop the tomatoes and add to the pan.

4. Add the tomato *purée*, herbs, and sugar. Heat and stir for about 10 minutes.

5. Season to taste. Serve hot.

Note: See recipe (page 68) for Cod Portugaise which uses this sauce.

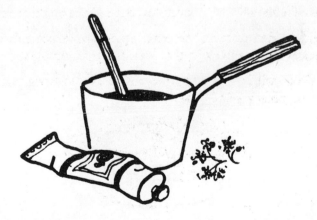

GRILLED MEAT

Grilling steak (beef), veal, lamb or pork makes a quick and easy meat course. Steaks, chops or fillets can be rubbed with a cut clove of garlic or sprinkled with herbs for variety. Grill on both sides for a few minutes until tender.

Here are some serving suggestions:

Grilled steak with fried mushrooms and onions.
Lamb chops rubbed with garlic and sprinkled with rosemary.
Pork chops with stewed apple (as apple sauce)
Lamb chops sprinkled with dried tarragon and served with grilled tomatoes.

See recipe for mint sauce (page 88) to serve with plain grilled lamb chops. Stir-fry is also a good vegetable dish to serve with grilled meat.

Good accompaniments are grilled tomatoes, fried mushrooms and onions, green vegetables and potatoes or plain boiled rice.

NUT ROAST
(Serves 2)

Imperial (Metric)	American
1 onion peeled and chopped	1 onion peeled and chopped
1 slice wheat-free bread, made into crumbs	1 slice wheat-free bread, made into crumbs
3 teaspoonsful wheat-free soya sauce	3 teaspoonsful wheat-free soy sauce
1 heaped teaspoonful tomato *purée*	1 heaped teaspoonful tomato paste
3 tinned tomatoes, chopped	3 canned tomatoes, chopped
1 grated eating apple	1 grated eating apple
3 oz (75g) ground hazelnuts	¾ cupful ground hazelnuts
3 good pinches dried mixed herbs	3 good pinches dried mixed herbs
Sea salt	Sea salt
Freshly ground black pepper	Freshly ground black pepper
Oil for greasing	Oil for greasing

1. Mix the first eight ingredients in a bowl.

2. Season.

3. Grease a shallow ovenproof dish. Turn the mixture into this. Flatten with a knife.

4. Bake in a preheated oven 425°F/220°C (Gas Mark 7), for about 25 minutes on the top shelf.

5. Serve with green vegetables and either potato or rice, plain boiled.

NUT RISSOLES
(Makes 5 to 6)

Make the recipe for Nut Roast but instead of turning into a dish shape make into flat cakes. Roll in maize flour (cornstarch) to coat and fry in shallow hot oil for about 3 minutes each side. Serve hot.

Note: Nut roasts and rissoles are usually bound with egg to stop them disintegrating. You will find that grated apple does this job just as well. A really delicious and light protein dish. For variety try ground cashews or walnuts, almonds or Brazils, or any mixture. A level tablespoonful freshly chopped parsley can be used instead of the dried herbs. Serve to the whole family.

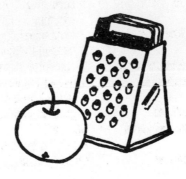

GRAVY

For people who have allergies the complexities of gravy mixes and
stock cubes are definitely out. The best approach is to make gravy
using the natural juices from grilled or roasted meat, thickened with
maize flour (cornmeal) and any vegetable strainings available. To
strengthen the stock a little wheat-free (thin) soya sauce can be added.
If you prefer, add a mashed boiled potato for thickening.

1. Strain off and discard the fat from meat juices left in the grill
    pan or roasting tin. It is important to do this well or the gravy
    will be too greasy.

2. Add the thickening of your choice and rub into the pan with the
    back of a wooden spoon. This will release any solid juices from
    the pan/tin as well as distribute the thickening.

3. Heat and cook while you add vegetable strainings or water.

4. Add the wheat-free soya sauce — 2 or 3 teaspoonsful to taste.

5. Bring to the boil and simmer for a couple of minutes. Serve hot.

LIVER WITH ORANGE AND BACON

Imperial (Metric)	American
2 oz (50g) lamb's liver	1 medium piece lamb's liver
Lean meat from 1 back rasher, chopped	Lean meat from 1 back rasher, chopped
1 tablespoonful vegetable oil	1 tablespoonful vegetable oil
½ a peeled orange, cut into slices	½ a peeled orange, cut into slices
2 teaspoonsful wheat-free soya sauce	2 teaspoonsful wheat-free soy sauce
1 tablespoonful pure orange juice	1 tablespoonful pure orange juice

1. Cut out any stringy pieces from the liver. Wash, dry and cut into
    small pieces.

2. Heat the oil in a frying pan (skillet) and put in the liver and bacon. Fry gently while turning to cook evenly for 5 minutes.

3. Put in the orange slices, soya sauce and orange juice. Heat through gently.

4. Serve hot with green vegetables and either plain boiled brown rice or potatoes.

Variation: If you prefer a thicker gravy dip the liver pieces in maize flour (cornmeal) before frying. (Seasoning is added at the table.)

KEBABS

This is a quick way of cooking food for a special dieter when the rest of the family is having quite a different meal. It is also an easy dish to take with you if going to someone else's home for a meal. All the hostess has to do is grill it for you, saving both of you worry and trouble.

Basically kebabs are small portions of fish, meat and vegetables grilled on a long skewer. Variations are endless and they look most attractive. When grilled they can be served on a bed of plain boiled brown rice.

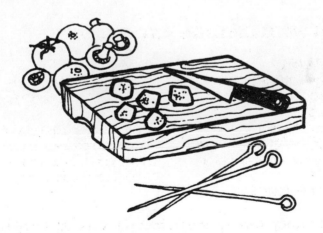

PORK KEBABS

Imperial (Metric)	American
2 oz (50g) trimmed pork fillet	1 medium-sized piece trimmed pork fillet
4 cubes of pineapple or pieces of apple	4 cubes of pineapple or pieces of apple
¼ of a green pepper, de-seeded, cut into 4 pieces	1 medium tomato, cut into 4
1 medium tomato, cut into 4	2 medium button mushrooms
2 medium button mushrooms	¼ of a green pepper, de-seeded, cut into 4 pieces
Vegetable oil	Vegetable oil
Sea salt and freshly ground black pepper	Sea salt and freshly ground black pepper

1. Cut the meat into about 4 or 5 pieces.

2. Assemble on 2 skewers, putting the pineapple next to the meat and the various vegetables etc. in between.

3. Brush with oil, season and grill, turning to ensure even cooking.

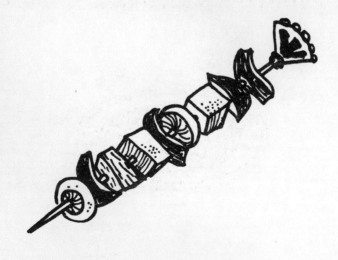

LAMB KEBABS

Imperial (Metric)	American
2 oz (50g) trimmed lamb from a chump chop, cut into 4 pieces	1 medium-sized piece of lamb from a chump chop, cut into 4 pieces
2 small tomatoes, cut in half	4 fresh mint leaves
2 button mushrooms, cut in half	2 small tomatoes, cut in half
4 fresh mint leaves	2 button mushrooms, cut in half
¼ of a red pepper, de-seeded and cut into 4	¼ of a red pepper, de-seeded and cut into 4

1. Assemble on 2 skewers, putting the mint leaves next to the meat, and the vegetables in between.

2. Brush with oil, season and grill, turning to ensure even cooking.

Other items to use are:
Stoned prunes, soaked overnight.
Dried apricot halves, soaked for 3 or 4 hours.
Cubes of lamb's liver.
Pieces of prepared kidney.
Cubes of grilling steak, trimmed of fat.
Cubes of cod fillet and thick slices of lemon.

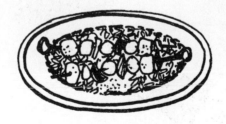

SAVOURY RICE

Imperial (Metric)	American
1 medium onion, peeled and chopped	1 medium onion, peeled and chopped
1 tablespoonful sunflower oil or similar	1 tablespoonful sunflower oil or similar
1 mushroom, chopped	1 mushroom, chopped
½ a red pepper, de-seeded and chopped	½ a red pepper, de-seeded and chopped
1 carrot, scrubbed and chopped	1 carrot, scrubbed and chopped
1 stick of celery, washed and chopped	1 stalk of celery, washed and chopped
2 tender cabbage or spinach leaves, shredded after trimming	2 tender cabbage or spinach leaves, shredded after trimming
1 portion cooked brown rice	1 portion cooked brown rice
Sea salt and freshly ground black pepper to taste	Sea salt and freshly ground black pepper to taste

1. Fry the onion gently in the oil for a few minutes.

2. Add the prepared vegetables and a little water to prevent sticking.

3. Cook with the lid on tightly for about 6 or 7 minutes.

4. Add the cooked rice and mix everything together. Cook until the rice has heated through.

5. Season and add the lemon juice, if liked.

6. Serve hot with fish or meat.

Variation: Other kinds of vegetables can be used according to season — green beans, peas, turnips, parsnips, broad beans (Windsor beans) etc. If you want to use tomato this is best served as a garnish as it is very soft when cooked and tends to make the dish too moist. If serving with fish sprinkle with a little fresh lemon juice. If serving with meat sprinkle with a little chopped (fresh) parsley.

PRAWN SAVOURY

Make Savoury Rice and add 1 heaped tablespoonful of peeled prawns for each person. Garnish with lemon.

SAVOURY RICE WITH BACON

Make Savoury Rice. For each person grill one rasher of back bacon. Remove and discard fat and chop remainder into small pieces. Add to the savoury rice and serve hot.

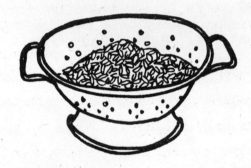

CHICKEN CURRY
(Serves 1)

This is a good meal to take with you when you are to eat in someone else's home, so saving the hostess worry of cooking two separate meals. Either get her to provide you with plain boiled rice or take your own. To make a richer stock add tomato juice instead of water.

Imperial (Metric)	American
½ a medium onion, peeled and sliced	½ a medium onion, peeled and sliced
2 teaspoonsful vegetable oil	2 teaspoonsful vegetable oil
1 mushroom, sliced	1 mushroom, sliced
2 tomatoes, chopped	2 tomatoes, chopped
2 teaspoonsful wheat-free soya sauce	2 teaspoonsful wheat-free soy sauce
1 boned chicken breast or 2 legs (unboned)	1 boned chicken breast or 2 legs (unboned)
1 heaped teaspoonful wheat-free curry powder	1 heaped teaspoonful wheat-free curry powder
Sea salt	Sea salt
Sprinkling of sultanas or raisins	Sprinkling of golden seedless raisins or raisins
½ an eating apple, cored and sliced	½ an eating apple, cored and sliced
Water	Water
1 heaped teaspoonful maize flour	1 heaped teaspoonful cornmeal

1. Cook the onion in the oil in a flameproof casserole, frying for about 4 minutes.

2. Add the mushrooms, tomatoes and soya sauce.

3. Put in the chicken and cook for about 2 minutes on each side to seal.

4. Sprinkle in the curry powder, salt to taste, the dried fruit and the apple slices.

5. Pour in enough water to cover and bring to the boil. Simmer gently with the lid on for about 45 minutes.

6. Mix the maize flour (cornmeal) with a little water and pour into the casserole. Stir until it thickens.

7. Serve on a bed of hot brown rice, plain boiled.

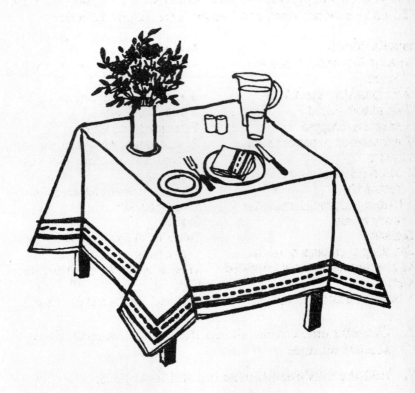

CHICKEN AND HERB CASSEROLE

This is an easy meal for one person and useful if the rest of the family is to eat something different.

Imperial (Metric)
½ medium onion, peeled and sliced
2 teaspoonsful vegetable oil
2 mushrooms, sliced
1 carrot, scrubbed and sliced
1 small tin tomatoes
2 teaspoonsful wheat-free soya sauce
1 boned chicken breast
1 large potato, peeled and sliced thinly
2 pinches of dried rosemary or 3 pinches of dried tarragon
Sea salt and freshly ground black pepper

American
½ medium onion, peeled and sliced
2 teaspoonsful vegetable oil
2 mushrooms, sliced
1 carrot, scrubbed and sliced
1 small can tomatoes
2 teaspoonsful wheat-free soy sauce
1 boned chicken breast
1 large potato, peeled and sliced thinly
2 pinches of dried rosemary or 3 pinches of dried tarragon
Sea salt and freshly ground black pepper

1. Preheat the oven to 400°F/200°C (Gas Mark 6).

2. Fry the onion in the oil until transparent.

3. Add the mushrooms, carrot, tomatoes and soya sauce.

4. Transfer to a warmed casserole. Stir and lay the chicken breast in the centre.

5. Cover with layers of the potato.

6. Season with salt and pepper and sprinkle with the chosen herb.

7. Put the lid on and bake for about an hour.

8. Spoon on to a warmed plate and serve.

Note: Serve this casserole with a green vegetable such as spinach, beans, fresh peas, sprouts or cabbage, lightly cooked. Alternatively offer a green salad as a side dish. Follow with a fruit salad for an easy but well balanced meal.

LEMON CHICKEN
(Serves 2-3)

This is a spicy Chinese dish. Serve with plain, boiled brown rice.

Imperial (Metric)	American
1 tablespoonful sherry	1 tablespoonful sherry
2 spring onions	2 scallions
1 small piece root ginger	1 small piece root ginger
3 portions cooked chicken, boned and trimmed	3 portions cooked chicken, boned and trimmed
1 tablespoonful sunflower or soya oil	1 tablespoonsful sunflower or soy oil
1 stick celery	1 stalk celery
2 medium mushrooms	2 medium mushrooms
½ medium green pepper	½ medium green pepper
1 tablespoonful wheat-free soya sauce (thin)	1 tablespoonful wheat-free soy sauce (thin)
Rind of 1 lemon	Rind of 1 lemon

1. Put the sherry into a basin.

2. Chop the spring onion (scallion), peel and shred the ginger and add to the sherry.

3. Mix in the chicken, cut into small pieces. Leave for about 20 minutes so that the chicken will absorb the flavour of the sherry etc.

4. Put the oil in a deep frying pan (skillet).

5. Chop the celery, slice the mushrooms and green pepper. Fry in the oil while you stir for about 2 minutes.

6. Add the chicken mixture and continue cooking for 2 more minutes.

7. Lastly, stir in the soya sauce and lemon rind (coarsely grated).

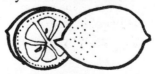

CHINESE FRIED RICE
(Serves 2)

Imperial (Metric)

1 generous tablespoonful sunflower or soya oil
2 spring onions, chopped
3 or 4 mushrooms, sliced
1 slice cooked ham, trimmed of fat and diced
2 heaped tablespoonsful cooked, peeled prawns
6 oz (150g) cooked long-grain brown rice
2 teaspoonsful wheat-free soya sauce
2 heaped tablespoonsful cooked, diced vegetables

American

1 generous tablespoonful sunflower or soy oil
2 scallions, chopped
3 or 4 mushrooms, sliced
1 slice cooked ham, trimmed of fat and diced
2 heaped tablespoonsful cooked, peeled prawns
1 cupful cooked long-grain brown rice
2 teaspoonsful wheat-free soy sauce
2 heaped tablespoonsful cooked, diced vegetables

1. Heat the oil in a deep frying pan (skillet).

2. Put in the onions and mushrooms and fry while you stir for 3 or 4 minutes.

3. Add all remaining ingredients and stir-fry for another 4 or 5 minutes.

4. Serve hot.

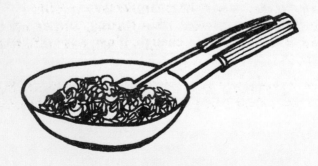

SWEET AND SOUR FISH
(Serves 2)

Imperial (Metric)	American
1 heaped tablespoonful maize flour	1 heaped tablespoonful cornstarch
2 portions cod fillets, cut into cubes	2 portions cod fillets, cut into cubes
Vegetable oil for frying	Vegetable oil for frying
1 onion, peeled and sliced	1 onion, peeled and sliced
4 mushrooms, sliced	4 mushrooms, sliced
3 tablespoonsful tomato juice	3 tablespoonsful tomato juice
1 tablespoonful wine vinegar	1 tablespoonful wine vinegar
2 teaspoonsful raw cane sugar	2 teaspoonsful raw cane sugar
2 tablespoonsful water	2 tablespoonsful water
1 tablespoonful maize flour for sauce	1 tablespoonful cornstarch for sauce

1. Put the heaped tablespoonful maize flour (cornstarch) into a paper bag and put in a few of the fish cubes. Close the bag and shake well to coat fish all over. Continue until all the cubes are coated.

2. Heat some oil — about a tablespoonful will do — in a small saucepan and put in the onion. Fry for 3 or 4 minutes. Put in the mushrooms and fry for another 3 minutes. Transfer to a dish and keep hot while you fry the fish.

4. Fry the coated fish cubes in hot oil until golden brown. Add to the onion/mushrooms and keep warm, in a bowl or dish.

5. In a small saucepan, mix the tomato juice, vinegar, sugar, water and maize flour (cornstarch) to make the sauce. Stir well and heat to boiling point. Simmer, while stirring, to make a thick sauce. Taste to see if it is sweet enough. If not, add a little more of the sugar.

6. Serve immediately with plain boiled rice and stir-fry vegetables. The sauce should be poured over the fish/mushrooms.

BEEF CASSEROLE WITH ORANGE
(Serves 2-3)

(Use a flameproof casserole.)

Imperial (Metric)	American
1 heaped tablespoonful maize flour	1 heaped tablespoonful cornmeal
Sea salt and freshly ground black pepper	Sea salt and freshly ground black pepper
¾ lb (350g) braising beef, trimmed and cut into small cubes	12 ounces braising beef, trimmed and cut into small cubes
1 medium onion, peeled and sliced	1 medium onion, peeled and sliced
½ a green pepper, de-seeded and chopped	½ a green pepper, de-seeded and chopped
1 tablespoonful vegetable oil	1 tablespoonful vegetable oil
Grated rind and juice of 1 orange	Grated rind and juice of 1 orange
1 tablespoonful wheat-free soya sauce	1 tablespoonful wheat-free soy sauce
Water	Water
1 tablespoonful chopped fresh parsley to garnish	1 tablespoonful chopped fresh parsley to garnish

1. Put the maize flour (cornmeal) into a paper bag. Season with salt and pepper, then add the meat cubes and toss to coat.

2. Fry the onion and pepper in the oil until soft.

3. Add the meat and fry while turning to seal, until evenly browned.

4. Transfer to a casserole with a lid. Stir in the orange rind, juice and soya sauce.

5. Top up with water, bring to the boil and put on the lid.

6. Bake in a preheated oven at 325°F/170°C (Gas Mark 3) for about 1½ hours.

7. Serve hot, sprinkled with parsley and accompanied by baked jacket potatoes and green vegetables.

ONION AND POTATO BAKE
(Serves 4)

Imperial (Metric)
4 large potatoes, peeled
4 medium onions
2 oz (50g) milk-free margarine
1 heaped teaspoonful freshly
  chopped parsley

American
4 large potatoes, peeled
4 medium onions
¼ cupful milk-free margarine
1 heaped teaspoonful freshly
  chopped parsley

1. Cut each potato into 4 pieces and boil in salted water for about 15 minutes.

2. Strain and cool a little. Slice thickly.

3. Preheat oven at 400°F/200°C (Gas Mark 6).

4. Peel the onions and chop or slice thinly.

5. Melt the margarine in a frying pan (skillet) and fry the onion for about 3 or 4 minutes.

6. Put the potato slices into a hot dish and spread the onion mixture over the top.

7. Finish cooking in the oven on the top shelf for about another 30 minutes.

8. Serve straight from the oven, sprinkled with the parsley.

Note: This dish has a rather sweet taste on account of the slow cooking of the onions. Most people prefer it without seasoning. Good with salad and lean cold meat such as chicken or ham.

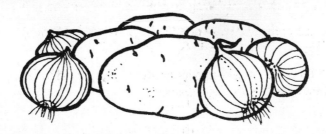

PORK CHOPS WITH APPLE SALAD
(Serves 2)

Imperial (Metric)	American
2 lean pork chops	2 lean pork chops
1 eating apple, grated (leave the skin on)	1 eating apple, grated (leave the skin on)
1 heaped teaspoonful sultanas	1 heaped teaspoonful golden seedless raisins
1 stick celery, chopped	1 stalk celery, chopped
6 lettuce leaves, torn into pieces	6 lettuce leaves, torn into pieces
2 tomatoes, sliced	2 tomatoes, sliced
Squeeze of fresh lemon juice	Squeeze of fresh lemon juice
Sprinkling of raw cane sugar	Sprinkling of raw cane sugar
Sea salt and freshly ground black pepper	Sea salt and freshly ground black pepper

1. Grill the pork chops on a metal grid — about 10 minutes each side.

2. Combine the apple, sultanas (golden seedless raisins), celery, lettuce and tomatoes in a bowl.

3. Sprinkle over the lemon juice and sugar. Season to taste.

4. Serve the chops on hot plates and the salad on side plates.

Note: Young, tender spinach leaves can be used instead of lettuce leaves.

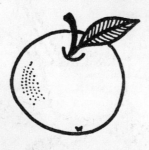

RISOTTO
(Serves 1)

Imperial (Metric)
1 small onion, chopped
1 teaspoonful sunflower or soya oil
2 mushrooms, sliced
1 portion cooked chicken, cut into
　　small pieces
Water
1 teaspoonful wheat-free soya sauce
6 oz (150g) cooked long-grain brown
　　rice
Sea salt and freshly ground black
　　pepper

American
1 small onion, chopped
1 teaspoonful sunflower or soy oil
2 mushrooms, sliced
1 portion cooked chicken, cut into
　　small pieces
Water
1 teaspoonful wheat-free soy sauce
1 cupful cooked long-grain brown
　　rice
Sea salt and freshly ground black
　　pepper

1. Fry the onion in the oil until transparent.

2. Put in the mushrooms and chicken, adding a little water to prevent sticking. Stir-fry for 3 or 4 minutes.

3. Add the soya sauce and the rice and stir well. Continue cooking while you stir for another 3 or 4 minutes.

4. Season to taste and serve hot accompanied by a green salad.

Note: This is a useful dish to take with you when going out to eat in someone else's house. It looks very appetizing and can be eaten hot or cold.

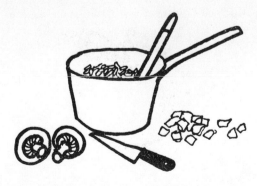

ROAST LAMB

Leg of lamb
Sea salt

1. Weigh the joint to find out how long it should be cooked for. Allow 20 minutes to the pound (per half kilo) and 20 minutes over.

2. Preheat oven at 425°F/220°C (Gas Mark 7).

3. Put the joint into a roasting tin, sprinkle with salt, put in the centre of the oven and cook for the amount of time you have calculated.

Note: Roast potatoes can be cooked at the same time on the top shelf. Serve with green vegetables in season and mint sauce. The gravy can be made from the meat juices left in the pan after straining off the fat.

MINT SAUCE

Imperial (Metric)	American
2 heaped tablespoonsful freshly chopped mint leaves	2 heaped tablespoonsful freshly chopped mint leaves
3 teaspoonsful raw cane sugar	3 teaspoonsful raw cane sugar
2 teaspoonsful boiling water	2 teaspoonsful boiling water
2 tablespoonsful wine vinegar	2 tablespoonsful wine vinegar

1. Put the chopped mint into a jug.

2. Add the sugar and mix well.

3. Add the boiling water which will help to dissolve the sugar.

4. Lastly, stir in the vinegar.

ROAST BEEF

Cook as for roast lamb but allow 15 minutes per pound (per half kilo) and 15 minutes over. If the joint is very lean you may need to spoon over a tablespoonful of sunflower or soya oil before cooking. This will give the traditional 'underdone' pink and red meat. If you prefer it well cooked, use the same instructions as for roast lamb. Serve with greens, roast potatoes and carrots or parsnips.

LIVER PROVENÇALE
(Serves 1)

Imperial (Metric)	American
4 oz (100g) lamb's liver	2 small pieces lamb's liver
Maize flour	Cornmeal
Sea salt and freshly ground black pepper	Sea salt and freshly ground black pepper
2 teaspoonsful sunflower or soya oil	2 teaspoonsful sunflower or soy oil
1 heaped teaspoonful milk-free margarine	1 heaped teaspoonful milk-free margarine
3 or 4 sprigs of fresh parsley, finely chopped	3 or 4 sprigs of fresh parsley, finely chopped
1 small clove garlic, crushed	1 small clove garlic, crushed
1 teaspoonful wine vinegar	1 teaspoonful wine vinegar

1. Trim the liver of all strings etc., and cut into thin slices.

2. Sprinkle with a little maize flour (cornmeal), salt and pepper.

3. Heat the oil in a small, heavy-based frying pan (skillet) and put in the slices of liver. Cook for about 1 minute each side.

4. Put on to a hot plate and keep warm.

5. Melt the knob of margarine in the frying pan (skillet) but do not let it brown.

6. Add the parsley and garlic and stir.

7. Add the vinegar, which will make it sizzle.

8. Pour over the liver and serve with mashed potatoes and hot vegetables or a green salad.

GOOD, OLD-FASHIONED STEW
(Serves 4 to 5)

This is a useful basic recipe because the whole course is cooked in one container. The vegetables can be varied according to what is in season or available — peas, broad beans, celery, green beans, turnips, parsnips, etc.

Imperial (Metric)

4 portions braising steak
Maize flour
4 onions, peeled and sliced
Sunflower oil
½ lb (¼ kilo) carrots, peeled and sliced
4 or 5 mushrooms, sliced
1 tablespoonful wheat-free soya sauce
Sea salt
Freshly ground black pepper
1 medium red or green pepper de-seeded and sliced
4 large potatoes (or equivalent) peeled if old and cut into 4
2 heaped tablespoonsful cooked beans — haricot, navy etc. (optional)
Extra vegetables in season

American

4 portions braising steak
Cornstarch
4 onions, peeled and sliced
Sunflower oil
½ pound carrots, peeled and sliced
4 or 5 mushrooms, sliced
1 tablespoonful wheat-free soy sauce
Sea salt
Freshly ground black pepper
1 medium red or green pepper de-seeded and sliced
4 large potatoes (or equivalent) peeled if old and cut into 4
2 heaped tablespoonsful cooked beans — haricot, navy etc. (optional)
Extra vegetables in season

1. Trim the meat of fat and gristle. Cut into cubes and roll in maize flour (cornstarch).

2. Fry the onion in a tablespoonful of sunflower oil, until it begins to brown, using a large saucepan or flameproof casserole.

3. Put in the meat cubes and another spoonful of oil. Fry while turning over, to seal the meat.

4. Add the soya sauce, all the vegetables (including the extras), the

beans if you are using them and enough water to cover.

5. Season. Bring to the boil while you stir. Transfer to a casserole
    if necessary and put into a preheated oven 425°F/220°C (Gas
    Mark 7), middle shelf. Cook for about 1 to 1¼ hours.

6. Serve hot with chunks of wheat-free bread for the special dieter
    and ordinary bread for the rest of the family.

Note: If the level of the liquid in the casserole goes too low, top up
with boiling water. Usually the potatoes will help to thicken the rich
gravy, but if you are using new ones that remain firm you may need
something more to thicken the gravy, e.g. put 1 tablespoonful of maize
flour (cornstarch) into a cup with 3 tablespoonsful water. Mix to a
smooth cream. Stir into the casserole. Cover again and put back into
the oven.

An ideal meal to save washing up and effort in the kitchen! It can
be served to the whole family and any leftovers can be reheated the
following day. A little wheat-free curry powder will make it into a
curry to be eaten with plain boiled rice.

In terms of nutritional value this recipe is worth a closer look. The
proportions of fat to protein to fibre are excellent providing the meat
is trimmed of all visible fat before cooking. Fats are both saturated
and unsaturated. None of the vegetables need to be strained so all
juices are eaten. It is not oversalted. Vegetables form the basis of the
dish and if these are all fresh so much the better. If served with a
dark green vegetable such as kale, broccoli or cabbage this dish is
really good. It is the kind of food that our great-grandparents would
have enjoyed — a simple, well balanced meal, easy to prepare,
nourishing and appetizing.

BOLOGNAISE SAUCE
(Serves 4 to 5)

Imperial (Metric)
1 tablespoonful sunflower oil
2 medium onions, peeled and sliced
 finely
2 rashers back bacon, trimmed of fat
2 oz (50g) chicken livers
½ lb (¼ kilo) minced beef (raw)
2 cloves garlic, peeled
2 level teaspoonsful maize flour
1½ pints (¾ litre) water
½ lb (¼ kilo) diced mixed
 vegetables
1 medium tin tomatoes, chopped
1 tablespoonful tomato *purée*
1 tablespoonful wheat-free soya
 sauce
A bouquet garni

American
1 tablespoonful sunflower oil
2 medium onions, peeled and sliced
 finely
2 rashers back bacon, trimmed of fat
½ cupful chicken livers
8 ounces minced beef (raw)
2 cloves garlic, peeled
2 level teaspoonsful cornstarch
3¾ cupsful water
8 ounces diced mixed vegetables
1 medium can tomatoes, chopped
1 tablespoonful tomato paste
1 tablespoonful wheat-free soy
 sauce
A bouquet garni

1. Heat the oil in a large pan. Fry the onions while stirring, until they are soft.

2. Cut the bacon into small squares. Cut out and discard the stringy parts of the livers and chop.

3. Add to the onion and fry gently while you stir for another couple of minutes.

4. Put in the minced beef and turn up the heat to fry briskly for about 3 minutes, turning the mixture over to brown the meats.

5. Peel the garlic. Crush into the meat mixture.

6. Mix the maize flour (cornstarch) in a cup with a little of the water. Add to the pan and stir.

7. Put in the vegetables, chopped tomatoes, tomato *purée* and soya sauce.

8. Pour in the remainder of the water and bring to the boil while stirring.

9. Season and add the bouquet garni.

10. Simmer for about 30 minutes, giving the occasional stir.

11. Take out the bouquet garni and serve hot with plain, boiled rice and a green side salad.

Note: The rich dark sauce complements the rice. Serve with mixed green side salad and follow with fruit for a balanced meal.

Vegetables for Main Meals

MASHED POTATOES

Boiled (floury) potatoes
Milk-free margarine
Hot water
Sea salt and freshly ground black pepper
Ground nutmeg

1. Mash the potatoes while still hot.

2. Add a knob of margarine for each portion and let it melt into the potato.

3. Beat in enough hot water to make the potatoes creamy.

4. Season to taste and add a small pinch of nutmeg for each portion.

5. Serve hot with a suitable meat or fish dish and vegetables.

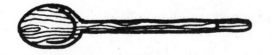

CRISPY ROAST POTATOES
Use old potatoes for this dish.

Potatoes, peeled and cut into even-sized pieces
Sunflower or soya oil
Sea salt

1. Preheat oven at 425°F/220°C (Gas Mark 7).

2. Cook the potatoes for 10 minutes in boiling water, then strain them.

3. Oil an ovenproof dish with the oil. Put the partly cooked potatoes into this and spoon a little oil over each potato.

4. Sprinkle with salt.

5. Bake on the top shelf for about an hour, turning the heat up slightly for the last 10 minutes to crisp them well.

6. Serve immediately.

SPINACH

Imperial (Metric)	American
½ lb (¼ kilo) fresh raw spinach per person	8 ounces fresh raw spinach per person
Sea salt	Sea salt
Water	Water

1. Fill the sink with cold water and wash spinach really well.

2. Tear off the green parts of the larger leaves and discard stalks.

3. Put into a large saucepan with a sprinkling of salt and 1 table-spoonful of water.

4. Put the lid on and cook gently for 10 to 15 minutes until tender. Poke the leaves down with a wooden spoon after the first 5 minutes.

5.   Drain well in a colander. Chop with a sharp knife and serve hot.

Note: Spinach contains a good deal of moisture and does not need to be cooked in water. The natural juices will run out of the leaves during cooking. The strainings can be used for enriching soup, gravy, etc.

ROOT VEGETABLES

Turnips, carrots, swede (rutabaga) and parsnips
Prepare by trimming and scrubbing, then cut into pieces and cook as follows:

1.   Put into a saucepan which has enough boiling, salted water to come halfway up the vegetables.

2.   Bring to the boil and simmer with the lid on until tender but not soft.

3.   Serve hot.

Note: Young vegetables will take only 20 to 25 minutes. Older vegetables may take a little longer. Parsnips can be roasted in the oven as for roast potatoes.

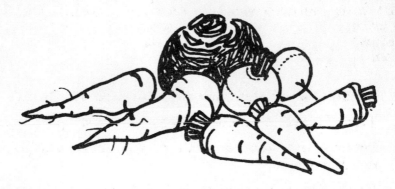

GREENS

Prepare by trimming off all discoloured leaves etc. On outside leaves, tear the leaf away from tough stalks and discard the latter. Sprouts should be trimmed at the base and cut into four.

After preparation and thorough washing, cook sprouts, cabbage, spring greens, sprout tops, kale and broccoli in the same way.

1. Put ¼ in. (5mm) water into a saucepan and bring to the boil.

2. Add a sprinkling of sea salt and put in the prepared greens, poking them down (leafy ones) with a wooden spoon.

3. Put the lid on and cook gently after bringing to the boil. Seven to 10 minutes should be ample.

4. Serve immediately.

Note: Many cooks start with good quality fresh greens and then ruin them by boiling in large quantities of water and by adding bicarbonate of soda (baking soda). Most of the goodness escapes into the water which is then thrown away, and the bicarbonate of soda (baking soda) finishes off most of the vitamins! (It is very important to eat at least one large portion of greens per day. They should be fresh and not frozen or tinned for maximum nutrition.)

BROAD BEANS (WINDSOR BEANS)

Shell and cook as for root vegetables.

CAULIFLOWER

Trim off tough outer leaves. Cut a slice off the root part at the base and discard. Wash thoroughly and cut into 6 or 8 sections, depending on size. Cook as for greens.

PEAS

Shell and cook as for greens.

GREEN BEANS

Cut off strings (if necessary) cut into short lengths. Cook as for greens.

STIR-FRY VEGETABLES

All vegetables can be cooked by the stir-fry method, which is not only quick but retains the maximum of vitamins and minerals possible for cooked vegetables.

1. Prepare a selection of vegetables including onion.

2. Cut into thin slices or shred, whichever is suitable.

3. Put a tablespoonful of sunflower or soya oil into a wok or deep frying pan (skillet) and heat.

4. Put in the onion and fry for a minute.

5. Gradually put in the vegetables, the hardest ones first (carrots, potatoes, turnips, etc.) and the softest last (tomatoes, cucumber, beansprouts, etc.). Stir-fry, turning the vegetables over gently and moving them to the outside of the pan as they become softened.

6. If the vegetables begin to stick, then add a little water.

The juices of all the vegetables will accumulate at the bottom of the pan. If you add 2 or 3 teaspoonsful of wheat-free soya sauce you will have a delicious gravy. (This way of cooking vegetables does not usually need seasoning.)

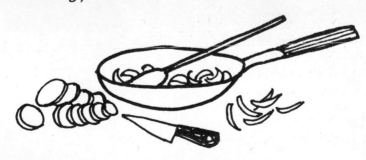

COLD MEAT AND SALADS

Beef, lamb and pork slices cut off a cold joint roasted the day before make an easy meal with salad and jacket potatoes. Here are some salad suggestions and instructions for the jacket potatoes.

SEASONAL SALADS

A healthy diet should contain a good portion of raw salad every day. This can be eaten with cold meat, fish or nuts and hot potatoes baked in their jackets, plain boiled or mashed.

Some cooked vegetables such as broad beans (Windsor beans), green beans and peas can be used to make a salad interesting. Brightly coloured vegetables such as carrot, tomatoes, red pepper and beetroot (beet) can also be used to add colour to the more dull-looking vegetables like swede (rutabaga), parsnip and white cabbage, etc.

Here are two lists of salad vegetables and fruit. Two items from each list, combined and dressed with either a lemon dressing or an oil and vinegar dressing, a sprinkling of sea salt, freshly ground black pepper and a little raw cane sugar (optional) will make interesting salads for one.

Soft/moist:

Cucumber, 1 in. (25mm) sliced or chopped
Spring onion (scallion), chopped small
Cooked green beans, 2 heaped tablespoonsful
Cooked broad beans (Windsor beans), 1 heaped tablespoonful
Peas, cooked, 2 heaped tablespoonsful
Raw mushrooms, 2 medium-sized, chopped or sliced
Eating apple, ½ a medium fruit, grated or sliced, skin left on
Grapes, 6 to 8 de-pipped
¼ peeled orange, sliced
½ tangerine, satsuma or clementine, divided into segments
Sultanas (golden seedless raisins) or raisins, 1 tablespoonful
Cold cooked haricot (dried) or butter (Lima) beans, 1 heaped tablespoonful
1 tomato, sliced

Crisp/crunchy:

Carrot, 1 small grated
Raw peas, 1 heaped tablespoonful
Parsnip, ½ medium-sized, grated coarsely
Swede (rutabaga) or beetroot (beet) 1 in. (25mm) cubes or grated
¼ green, red or yellow pepper, chopped
Watercress, ¼ of a bunch of sprigs
Lettuce, 4 leaves
Cress, ½ packet
Spinach or curly kale, 3 young leaves, shredded
Brussels sprouts, 4 shredded
Cabbage, 1 portion of red, green or white, shredded finely
Cauliflower, 4 florets
Beansprouts, 2 heaped tablespoonsful, chopped or left whole
Celery, 1 stalk, chopped or sliced

LEMON DRESSING

Imperial (Metric)	American
1 tablespoonful fresh lemon juice	1 tablespoonful fresh lemon juice
3 tablespoonsful sunflower or soya oil	3 tablespoonsful sunflower or soy sauce
1 teaspoonful raw cane sugar	1 teaspoonful raw cane sugar
Sea salt and freshly ground black pepper to taste	Sea salt and freshly ground black pepper to taste

1. Put all ingredients into a screw-top jar.

2. Shake vigorously to combine before sprinkling over salads.

Note: This dressing has a very fresh taste. It is especially good for salads which contain apple, raw mushrooms and cooked peas as the lemon will stop them turning brown or yellow.

RICE SALAD
(Serves 1)

Imperial (Metric)	American
2 heaped tablespoonsful cooked brown rice	2 heaped tablespoonsful cooked brown rice
1 spring onion	1 scallion
1 heaped tablespoonful chopped red pepper	1 heaped tablespoonful chopped red pepper
Sprinkle of sultanas	Sprinkle of golden seedless raisins
1 tablespoonful cold cooked peas	1 tablespoonful cold cooked peas
2 or 3 walnuts, chopped	2 or 3 English walnuts, chopped
1 small mushroom, chopped	1 small mushroom, chopped
1 tablespoonful sunflower oil	1 tablespoonful sunflower oil
2 teaspoonsful lemon juice	2 teaspoonsful lemon juice
Sea salt	Sea salt
Freshly ground black pepper	Freshly ground black pepper
Raw cane sugar	Raw cane sugar

1. Put the first seven ingredients into a small bowl.

2. Mix well.

3. Put the sunflower oil and lemon juice into a cup and mix with a teaspoon.

4. Season with the salt and pepper and enough sugar to make a slightly sweet dressing.

5. Dress the salad and serve immediately with cold meat or fish.

Note: If you wish to garnish the salad use a slice of lemon and a sprig of parsley.

OIL AND VINEGAR DRESSING

Put 1 tablespoonful of wine or cider vinegar and 3 tablespoonsful of sunflower oil into a screw-top jar. Shake well before using. (This dressing should be used to moisten salads not to swamp them.)

MINTY DRESSING

Imperial (Metric)
1 teaspoonful freshly chopped mint leaves
1 teaspoonful French mustard (wheat-free)
2 teaspoonsful lemon juice
2 teaspoonsful finely chopped onion or chives
Raw cane sugar or fructose

American
1 teaspoonful freshly chopped mint leaves
1 teaspoonful French mustard (wheat-free)
2 teaspoonsful lemon juice
2 teaspoonsful finely chopped onion or chives
Raw cane sugar or fructose

1. Put the first four ingredients into a screw-top jar and put the top on. Shake vigorously to combine.

2. Taste and add raw cane sugar or fructose to taste. Shake again.

Note: Use leftover cold, boiled new potatoes and peas. Serve with cold roast lamb and salad.

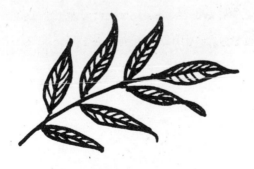

FRENCH DRESSING
(Makes about ¼ pint/150ml)

Imperial (Metric)
2 tablespoonsful white wine vinegar
6 tablespoonsful sunflower oil
1 teaspoonful French Mustard
  (wheat-free)
½ clove garlic, peeled and crushed
1 teaspoonful raw cane sugar or
  fructose
Sea salt and freshly ground black
  pepper

American
2 tablespoonsful white wine vinegar
6 tablespoonsful sunflower oil
1 teaspoonful French Mustard
  (wheat-free)
½ clove garlic, peeled and crushed
1 teaspoonful raw cane sugar or
  fructose
Sea salt and freshly ground black
  pepper

1. Put the first five ingredients into a screw-top jar.

2. Add seasoning to taste.

3. Put on the top and shake well until all ingredients have combined.

4. Store in the fridge and use as required. Always shake well before using.

JACKET POTATOES
Choose old potatoes and scrub with a hard brush to remove any dirt. Cut out any 'eyes' or discoloured parts with a sharp knife. Pierce the skin with the point of the knife in several places. (This is to let out steam during baking.) Put a metal skewer through the centre of each one and place on a baking sheet. Bake in a preheated oven at 425°F/220°C (Gas Mark 7) for about an hour or until the flesh is soft. Eat the whole potato including the skin and serve with milk-free margarine.

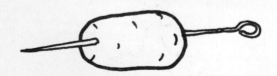

12.
PUDDINGS

The items you will miss on this special kind of diet are mainly the ones made with milk and eggs. You may not serve milk puddings or quick whipped desserts, ice cream or yogurt and so will have to rely rather heavily on fruit puddings. In its simplest form this type of pudding is really no trouble at all, cheap and high in vitamins. The seasons bring us a good variety of fruit and imports of more exotic kinds of fruit add even more interest and variety.

Use fresh fruit, not tinned or frozen, for maximum nutrition and flavour. The following may sound rather simple in the way of recipes but they are all delicious and easy to prepare. Remember, you may not have cream or custard so use only the best quality fruit.

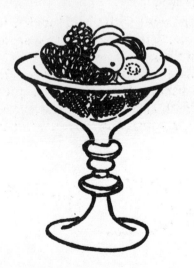

FRUIT SALAD

Fruit salad is always refreshing. Peel and slice fruits so that they are easy to eat. Sweeten to taste with a little raw cane sugar or honey and moisten with fresh orange juice. Try the following combinations for variety.

1 small eating pear, 3 or 4 peeled; de-stoned and sliced lychees, about 8 melon cubes — good to follow a Chinese main course;

1 small eating apple, 4 or 5 strawberries, a few melon cubes or banana slices;

½ kiwi fruit, peeled and sliced, ½ an orange, sliced, 5 or 6 seedless grapes;

1 fresh peach, peeled, stoned and sliced, a handful of raspberries or stoned, sweet cherries;

Orange and grapefruit slices mixed.

Some fruits are nicest eaten on their own, such as figs and nectarines, but the fruit must be really good or it will be a disappointment. Serve strawberries or raspberries with a little raw cane sugar. Merely wash the fruit and remove the hulls. Serve in a glass dish. There are many varieties of apples and pears in the shops, as well as plums, grapes and soft fruits such as peaches and apricots.

The more sour types of fruit can be stewed and sweetened with raw cane sugar or honey. Apples, cooking pears, plums, apricots, gooseberries, black and redcurrants, peaches, damsons and greengages.

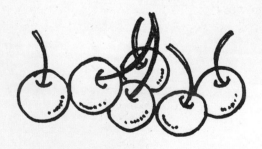

STEWED FRUIT

1. Prepare the fruit — either a single type of fruit or a mixture.

2. Cut into pieces or slices and put into a saucepan with a little water and sugar to taste.

3. Bring slowly to the boil and then simmer until tender.

4. Serve hot or cold.

Some fruit contains more moisture than others. Rhubarb can be stewed without any water at all provided you stir while it cooks. Apples and plums need very little water.

Good mixtures are:

a. **Apple and rhubarb**

b. **Apple and blackcurrant**

c. **Peach and redcurrant**

d. **Plum and pear**

e. **Peach and raspberry**

f. **Apricot and raspberry**

At the end of the soft fruit season and when prices are low because of a glut or an extra good crop, try a *compote* of apple, pear, plum, blackcurrant, redcurrant, plum, damson, etc., as available.

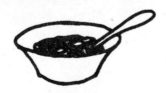

JAM TARTS

Imperial (Metric)	American
4 oz (100g) *Trufree* No. 6 plain flour	½ cupful *Trufree* No. 6 plain flour
2 pinches of sea salt	2 pinches of sea salt
1½ oz (40g) milk-free margarine	¼ cupful milk-free margarine
About 3 tablespoonsful cold water	About 3 tablespoonsful cold water
Raw sugar jam	Raw sugar jelly

1. Preheat oven at 425°F/220°C (Gas Mark 7).

2. Mix the flour and salt in a mixing bowl.

3. Rub in the margarine until the mixture resembles fine breadcrumbs.

4. Add the water and mix to a sticky paste.

5. Knead into one ball of dough using a little more of the flour.

6. Roll out as for ordinary pastry and cut into 6 rounds with a pastry cutter.

7. Using round patty tins (with curved and not straight sides), lift the rounds into these with a spatula. Press down into the tins with the knuckle of your forefinger.

8. Fill each tart with a teaspoonful of jam.

9. Bake on the top shelf for about 20 minutes.

10. Serve hot for a pudding or cold for tea or a snack.

Note: Use this pastry for mince pies, apple tartlets, etc.

N.B. If *Trufree* flour is unobtainable, use the recipe for pastry in Fruit Tart with Nuts. This is a blending of ground rice, milk-free margarine and grated apple.

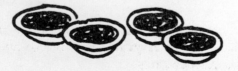

APRICOT TART WITH NUTS
A refreshing pudding that can be served all the year round, hot or cold.

Pastry:

Imperial (Metric)	American
2 oz (50g) milk-free margarine	¼ cupful milk-free margarine
4 oz (100g) ground brown rice	½ cupful brown rice
3 oz (75g) grated eating apple	1 small eating apple, grated

Filling:

6 oz (150g) dried apricots	1 cupful dried apricots
2 heaped teaspoonsful raw cane sugar	2 heaped teaspoonsful raw cane sugar
½ pint (¼ litre) cold water	1⅓ cupsful cold water
2 teaspoonsful fresh lemon juice	2 teaspoonsful fresh lemon juice
1 oz (25g) chopped, shelled nuts	¼ cupful chopped, shelled nuts

1. Preheat oven at 425°F/220°C (Gas Mark 7).

2. Pick over and wash apricots before chopping into small pieces.

3. Put into a saucepan with the sugar, water and lemon juice. Bring to the boil and simmer until all the water has been absorbed.

4. Use a fork to blend the margarine, ground rice and apple. Knead until one ball of dough is formed.

5. Grease an enamel pie-plate and put the dough in the centre. Flatten with the palm and fingers until it has spread evenly over the plate. Raise a slight edge all the way round with the fingers.

6. Spread the filling evenly over the pastry and sprinkle with the nuts.

7. Bake for 20 to 25 minutes on the top shelf and serve hot or cold in slices.

Variation: If preferred sprinkle with a mixture of sunflower seeds and sesame seeds instead of the nuts. A sprinkle of powdered cinnamon in the pastry will make this tart spicy.

BANANA FRITTERS
(Serves 4)

Imperial (Metric)	American
2 oz (50g) potato flour (farina)	1/3 cupful potato flour (farina)
1/2 teaspoonful dried apple pectin	1/2 teaspoonful dried apple pectin
1 tablespoonful soya flour	1 tablespoonful soy flour
5 tablespoonsful cold water	5 tablespoonsful cold water
2 medium bananas	2 medium bananas
Sunflower oil or similar for frying	Sunflower oil or similar for frying
Raw cane sugar for sprinkling	Raw cane sugar for sprinkling

1. Put a serving plate to warm.

2. Mix the potato flour, pectin, soya flour and cold water in a bowl. Beat to a creamy batter.

3. Peel and core the apples and cut into wedges — each one should make 8 wedges.

4. Dip these in the batter so that they are evenly coated all over.

5. Fry in shallow, hot oil, turning once, until brown. This will take about a minute each side.

6. Serve on warmed plates sprinkled with a little sugar.

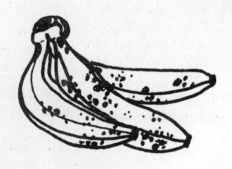

FRUIT AND NUT CRUNCH
(Serves 2)

Imperial (Metric)	American
1 generous knob milk-free margarine	1 generous knob milk-free margarine
1 slice wheat-free bread	1 slice wheat-free bread
3 teaspoonsful raw cane sugar	3 teaspoonsful raw cane sugar
1 tablespoonful hazelnuts, chopped and roasted	1 tablespoonful hazelnuts, chopped and roasted
1 portion stewed apricots	1 portion stewed apricots

1. Melt the margarine in a small frying pan (skillet).

2. Add the breadcrumbs and fry until golden and crisp.

3. Leave to cool and then stir in the sugar and nuts.

4. Put a layer of the fruit in a large wine glass.

5. Sprinkle with a layer of the crunch mixture.

6. Spoon on another layer of the fruit, using it all up.

7. Finish with the rest of the crunch mixture and flatten.

This recipe can be varied in several ways. Any kind of stewed fruit can be used provided it is not too watery (e.g. rhubarb would be too liquid). Try apple, pear, peach, cherries, or mixtures such as blackberry and apple. Fresh fruit can also be used — pineapple, fresh ripe peach, strawberries, raspberries or any such mixture. Banana can also be used, cut into thin slices and with a little orange juice poured over to moisten it. Any chopped and roasted nuts can be used such as almonds and walnuts. If you cannot buy these already roasted, chop and then dry out in a very low oven for about 20 minutes. If in a hurry put under a medium grill for about 10 minutes.

Note: Although this sweet is crunchiest served cold it can be served hot too. (Both the crunch and the fruit should be hot.)

STUFFED PEACHES
(Serves 1)

Imperial (Metric)	American
1 large, firm peach	1 large, firm peach
1 oz (25g) wheat-free crumbs*	1 heaped tablespoonful wheat-free crumbs*
3 teaspoonsful raw cane sugar	3 teaspoonsful raw cane sugar
1 heaped teaspoonful ground almonds	1 heaped teaspoonful ground almonds
3 heaped teaspoonsful milk-free margarine	3 heaped teaspoonsful milk-free margarine
Sprinkle of grated lemon rind	Sprinkle of grated lemon rind
Flaked almonds to decorate	Slivered almonds to decorate

1. Preheat oven at 350°F/180°C (Gas Mark 4).

2. Wash the peach and remove stone. Scoop a little flesh from around the centre and put into a cup.

3. Add the crumbs, sugar, ground almonds, margarine and lemon rind. Beat to a cream with a small spoon. If the mixture is too stiff add a little water.

4. Divide between the two peach halves and stuff the cavity left by the stone.

5. Put into a small oven-proof dish, greased with milk-free margarine. Sprinkle with flaked almonds.

6. Bake above centre of oven for about 25 to 30 minutes.

7. Serve hot or cold.

Note: This makes a nice treat for a special dieter and can be baked in the oven when other items are being baked for the rest of the family, or when special wheat-free bread is being baked on the same setting. A delicious way of using the not-so ripe peaches available from the fruiterer and supermarket.

* Any kind of plain cake such as sponge as long as it is wheat-free,

egg-free and milk-free — see recipes in this book.

RED FRUIT SALAD

Combine raspberries, strawberries, redcurrants cherries and blackberries in a dish, as available. Sprinkle with lemon juice and raw cane sugar to taste.

FRIED BANANAS
(Serves 1)

Imperial (Metric)	American
Generous knob of milk-free margarine	Generous knob of milk-free margarine
2 small or 1 large banana	2 small or 1 large banana
Fresh lemon juice	Fresh lemon juice
2 teaspoonsful brandy	2 teaspoonsful brandy
Raw cane sugar	Raw cane sugar

1. Melt the margarine in a smallish frying pan (skillet).

2. Peel the banana(s) and cut in half lengthways.

3. As soon as the margarine starts to foam put in the banana slices.

4. Brown on both sides over a gentle heat.

5. Squeeze in a little lemon juice (a rather sizzly affair!) and remove from heat.

6. Add the brandy, if using.

7. Sprinkle with the sugar and serve hot, immediately.

Note: This is a simple dish to be made at the last minute but it is quite delicious. A useful sweet for the special dieter when the rest of the family are having a different dish. Omit the brandy if serving to a child.

BAKED FRUIT

Fruit which has been baked in the oven tastes quite different from stewed fruit. Often, if the oven is already being used for another dish, it is easy to put in a dish of fruit to bake. If the oven is on a high heat put the fruit low down in the oven. If on a medium heat use the top of the oven.

Several kinds of fruit are suitable for baking — apples, rhubarb, apricots, peaches, plums, greengages, red and black currants, pears etc., or any mixture in season such as blackberry and apple. Fruit juice, water or wine can be used to keep the fruit moist. Here is a typical example of baked fruit:

Baked Apricots
1. Put 1½ lbs (675g) of fresh, washed apricots, in an ovenproof dish.
2. Sprinkle with raw cane sugar to taste and the juice of a lemon. Put on the lid.
3. Bake in a preheated oven 300°F/150°C (Gas Mark 2) for about ¾ hour to 1 hour or until the fruit is soft.
4. Serve hot or cold.

Baked Apples
If baking apples, leave the peel on but remove the central core. Cut a line round the 'waist'. Fill the centre with raisins or other fruit such as raspberries or blackberries. Sprinkle with a little raw cane sugar (or liquid honey) and bake in a dish with a little water until soft. This should take about half an hour at 350°F/180°C (Gas Mark 4). (No lid required).

Pears in Wine
Pears can be peeled and left whole. Cooked in red wine with a few pinches of cinnamon they make a delicious dessert.

Baked Bananas
Bananas require little cooking time and are best cooked in pineapple

or orange juice. Bake in a shallow dish at 350°F/180°C (Gas Mark 4) for a mere 15 minutes, top shelf. They can be sprinkled with chopped dates instead of a sweetener for variation. (No lid required).

FRUIT DESSERT

Imperial (Metric)
1 slightly heaped tablespoonful ground brown rice
¼ pint (150ml) unsweetened orange or pineapple juice
1 tablespoonful raw cane sugar
1 teaspoonful vegetable oil

American
1 slightly heaped tablespoonful ground brown rice
⅔ cupful unsweetened orange or pineapple juice
1 tablespoonful raw cane sugar
1 teaspoonful vegetable oil

1. Put all ingredients into a small saucepan and mix until smooth.

2. Heat to boiling point and cook, while stirring, for 2 minutes or until thick.

3. Leave to grow cold. Serve chilled from the fridge.

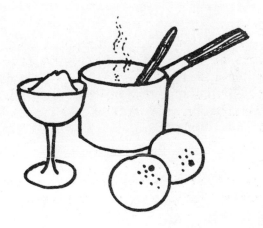

RICE AND SULTANA PUDDING

Imperial (Metric)
1 (½ litre) tablespoonful soya flour
1 pint (½ litre) water
1 oz (25g) milk-free margarine
3 tablespoonsful brown rice
   (uncooked)
2 tablespoonsful raw cane sugar
1 heaped tablespoonful sultanas
Few drops of pure vanilla flavouring
Grated nutmeg

American
1 tablespoonful soy flour
2½ cupsful water
2½ tablespoonsful milk-free
   margarine
3 tablespoonsful brown rice
   (uncooked)
2 tablespoonsful raw cane sugar
1 heaped tablespoonful golden
   seedless raisins
Few drops of pure vanilla flavouring
Grated nutmeg

1. Put the soya flour into a saucepan with a little of the water and mix until smooth.

2. Add the rest of the water and bring to the boil. Simmer for 5 minutes.

3. Add the margarine and stir until melted.

4. Put the rice and sugar into an ovenproof dish and pour the soya mixture over it.

5. Add the sultanas (golden seedless raisins) and vanilla flavouring. Stir well.

6. Sprinkle a little nutmeg over the top and bake for about 2½ hours at 275°F/140°C (Gas Mark 1). If it starts to dry out during cooking, add a little more (hot) water.

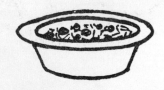

'CHEESE' AND BISCUITS

For people on a milk-free diet cheese is definitely out. However, the following recipe has a pleasant cheesy taste and looks very much like cheese spread.

Imperial (Metric)	American
4 teaspoonsful sunflower oil	4 teaspoonsful sunflower oil
3 pinches of sea salt	3 pinches of sea salt
½ clove garlic, peeled	½ clove garlic, peeled
1 oz (25g) ground almonds	¼ cupful ground almonds
About 8 drops of fresh lemon juice	About 8 drops of fresh lemon juice

1. Put the oil and salt into a small basin.

2. Rub the cut part of the garlic clove round the basin, spreading the oil and salt. Discard the clove.

3. Put in the ground almonds and mix with a fork to absorb the oil.

4. Add the lemon juice and mix to a paste.

5. Use as a spread on special wheat-free crispbreads or special wheat-free toast.

6. Serve with a crisp eating apple, pear, peach or nectarine and wheat-free crispbreads (page 34), water biscuits or sesame crackers (page 133).

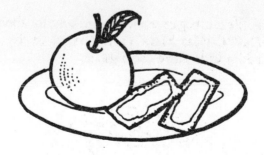

PINEAPPLE WATER ICE
(Serves 4)

Imperial (Metric)	American
1 small pineapple	1 small pineapple
8 oz (240ml) water	1⅓ cupsful water
1 tablespoonful lemon juice	1 tablespoonful lemon juice
Raw cane sugar to taste	Raw cane sugar to taste

1. Cut off the top and bottom of the pineapple. Trim off outside casing all round and discard. Also cut out the core and discard.

2. Cut flesh into dice and put into a saucepan with the water and lemon juice.

3. Bring to the boil and cook for about 5 minutes, adding sugar to taste.

4. Allow to cool a little and then blend in a liquidizer.

5. Spoon into a freezer container and freeze. Remove from freezer and then beat until the mixture becomes fluffy.

6. Freeze until needed.

Note: A light refreshing sweet that can be stored in the freezer and used as required.

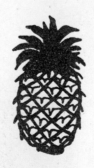

APRICOT AND HONEY DESSERT
(Serves 3)

This turns out as quite a creamy sweet yet no milk or cream are used.

Imperial (Metric)	American
4 oz (100g) dried apricots	¾ cupful dried apricots
Juice of ¼ of a lemon	Juice of ¼ of a lemon
Rind of ½ a lemon	Rind of ½ a lemon
1½ tablespoonsful liquid honey	1½ tablespoonsful liquid honey
¼ oz (7g) gelatine crystals	¼ oz gelatine crystals
2 tablespoonsful water (cold)	2 tablespoonsful water (cold)

1. Soak the apricots overnight in plenty of cold water.

2. The following day cook in a saucepan with enough water to cover. Bring to the boil and then simmer gently for 30 minutes or until the fruit is soft enough to *purée*.

3. Put the gelatine and water into a small basin over a pan of simmering water. Stir until dissolved and then mix in well with the apricots.

4. Put the apricots, lemon juice and rind into the blender with the honey. Liquidize.

5. Spoon into 3 glass dishes and leave to cool. Chill in the fridge until set.

6. Serve cold from the fridge.

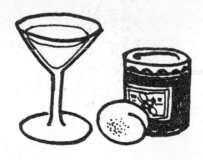

13.

TEAS AND TREATS

SULTANA SCONES
(Makes 8)

Imperial (Metric)
4 oz (100g) *Trufree* No. 4 or 5 flour
Pinch of sea salt
1 teaspoonful bicarbonate of soda
1 teaspoonful cream of tartar
1 oz (25g) milk-free margarine
1 oz (25g) raw cane sugar
1 oz (25g) sultanas
1 teaspoonful grated orange rind
Exactly 3 tablespoonsful cold water

American
1 cupful *Trufree* No. 4 or 5 flour
Pinch of sea salt
1 teaspoonful baking soda
1 teaspoonful cream of tartar
2½ tablespoonsful milk-free margarine
2½ tablespoonsful raw cane sugar
2½ tablespoonsful golden seedless raisins
1 teaspoonful grated orange rind
Exactly 3 tablespoonsful cold water

1. Preheat oven at 425°F/220°C (Gas Mark 7).

2. Put the flour, salt, bicarbonate of soda and cream of tartar into a bowl and mix thoroughly.

3. Add the margarine and rub it in with the fingers.

4. Stir in the sugar, fruit, rind and water.

5. Mix, then knead, to a soft dough using a little more of the flour if you need to.

6. Divide into 8 portions, roll into balls, flatten and then shape into scones.

7. Put on to a greased baking sheet and bake on the top shelf of the oven for 15-20 minutes.

8. Eat freshly baked, split and spread with milk-free margarine.

Note: If you prefer, roll the dough out and cut into rounds with a cutter.

FRUIT TRIFLE

Imperial (Metric)	American
1 sponge bun (see recipe, page 121)	1 sponge bun (see recipe, page 121)
Raw sugar red jam	Raw sugar red jelly
3 teaspoonsful fruit juice	3 teaspoonsful fruit juice
Slice of pineapple or ½ a peach	Slice of pineapple or ½ a peach
1 portion of Fruit Dessert (see recipe, page 113)	1 portion of Fruit Dessert (see recipe, page 113)
1 walnut and a sprinkling of blanched almonds to decorate	1 English walnut and a sprinkling of blanched almonds to decorate

1. Slice the bun in half and spread with the jam (jelly). Sandwich together and cut into pieces. Put in the bottom of an individual glass dish.

2. Spoon the fruit juice over the bun pieces.

3. Cut the fruit into pieces and place on top of the bun pieces.

4. Make the Fruit Dessert and spoon over the bun and fruit mixture.

5. Allow to cool and decorate with walnut (in the middle) and a sprinkling of blanched almonds.

Note: This is just as delicious and enviable as the ordinary kind of fruit trifle.

BROWN TEA BREAD

Imperial (Metric)
10¼ oz (290g) *Trufree* No. 5 flour
1 tablespoonful sunflower oil
1 sachet of yeast (provided with the flour)
8 fl oz (200ml) warm water
1 tablespoonful raw cane sugar
1 heaped tablespoonful raisins
1 heaped tablespoonful chopped walnuts
Grated rind of 1 orange

American
2½ cupsful *Trufree* No. 5 flour
1 tablespoonful sunflower oil
1 sachet of yeast (provided with the flour)
1 cupful warm water
1 tablespoonful raw cane sugar
1 heaped tablespoonful seedless raisins
1 heaped tablespoonful chopped English walnuts
Grated rind of 1 orange

1. Preheat oven at 350°F/180°C (Gas Mark 4).

2. Put the flour into a mixing bowl and sprinkle in the oil and yeast. Mix well.

3. Pour in the water and mix to a creamy batter.

4. Sprinkle in the sugar, fruit, nuts and rind. Mix well.

5. Spoon into a greased* 1 lb (½ kilo) loaf tin, size 6 × 3½ × 2¾ in. (15×9×7cm). Put immediately on to the top shelf of the oven and bake for about 1 hour.

6. Turn out of the tin carefully and cool on a wire rack. Do not cut until cold as this loaf needs to 'set'.

7. Store in a clean, sealed polythene bag.

Note: Although this loaf contains yeast it does not need to be left to rise. No kneading is required as the mixture is a kind of batter. The loaf will rise by about 50% during baking and should be brown and crusty.

Use for snacks or for tea sliced thickly and spread with milk-free margarine. Also good toasted the day after baking.

* Use milk-free margarine or cooking oil.

BASIC SPONGE MIX
(Enough for 6 buns)

Imperial (Metric)
½ oz (15g) soya flour
1 oz (25g) raw cane sugar
½ teaspoonful dried pectin
¾ oz (20g) potato flour (farina)
2 oz (50g) ground brown rice
½ oz (15g) yellow split pea flour
½ oz (15g) ground almonds
1 tablespoonful wheat-free and milk-free baking powder
5 tablespoonsful unsweetened orange juice
2 tablespoonsful sunflower oil or similar

American
1½ tablespoonsful soy flour
2½ tablespoonsful raw cane sugar
½ teaspoonful dried pectin
1½ tablespoonsful potato flour (farina)
¼ cupful ground brown rice
1 tablespoonful yellow split pea flour
1 tablespoonful ground almonds
1 tablespoonful wheat-free and milk-free baking soda
5 tablespoonsful unsweetened orange juice
2 tablespoonsful sunflower oil or similar

1. Preheat oven at 400°F/200°C (Gas Mark 6).

2. Put all ingredients into a bowl and mix with a wooden spoon until you have a creamy cake mix.

3. Put 6 cake (bun) papers into 6 patty tins, and spoon the cake mix into them.

4. Bake on the top shelf until golden — about 15 minutes.

5. Cool on a wire rack and eat on the day they are made. (Stale buns can be used in jelly, with fruit.)

Variation: For natural flavourings add either the grated rind of 1 orange or the grated rind of ½ a lemon.

Note: Most of the work in making these is in the weighing and measuring of the ingredients. See back of the book for details of the special baking powder or make your own. (See recipe, page 25.)

CAROB CAKE

Imperial (Metric)
1 oz (25g) soya flour
3 oz (50g) raw cane sugar
1½ teaspoonsful dried pectin
1 oz (25g) wheat-free carob powder
4 oz (100g) ground brown rice
¾ oz (20g) yellow split pea flour
1 oz (25g) finely ground nuts
2 heaped teaspoonsful special
   wheat-free and milk-free baking
   powder (see recipe, page 25)
¼ pint (150ml) orange juice
3 oz (75g) finely grated apple
2 tablespoonsful sunflower oil

American
¾ cupful soy flour
½ cupful raw cane sugar
1½ teaspoonsful dried pectin
¼ cupful carob powder (wheat-free)
½ cupful ground brown rice
1½ tablespoonsful yellow split pea
   flour
½ cupful finely ground nuts
2 heaped teaspoonsful special
   wheat-free and milk-free baking
   soda (see recipe, page 25)
⅔ cupful orange juice
1 small apple finely grated
2 tablespoonsful sunflower oil

1. Preheat oven at 400°F/200°C (Gas Mark 6).

2. Put all the ingredients into a bowl and mix to a cream.

3. Grease a tin size 7¼ × 3½ × 2¼ in. (185 × 90 × 60mm). Use milk-free margarine or sunflower oil. Flour with ground rice.

4. Spoon in the mixture and flatten with a knife.

5. Bake on the top shelf for about 45 to 50 minutes.

6. Turn out on to a wire rack to cool.

7. When quite cold, store in a sealed plastic bag.

8. Eat within 2 or 3 days.

Note: Use only dried pectin and not the liquid type used for making jams. Most of the work in this recipe is in the weighing out, which should be accurate and not guessed.

Variations:

Chocolate Cake
Use the Carob Cake recipe but substitute wheat-free cocoa powder for the carob.

Ginger Cake
Use the Carob Cake recipe but instead of carob add 2 heaped teaspoonsful ground ginger.

PARTY ALMONDS
Spread shelled almonds in a shallow baking tin and toast in a preheated oven at 300°F/150°C (Gas Mark 2) for about 20 minutes. Serve cold as a party nibble.

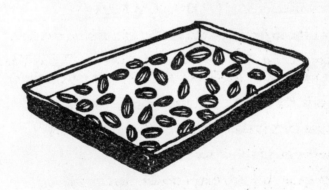

CELEBRATION FRUIT SALAD CAKE

Imperial (Metric)

2 oz (50g) soya flour
3 oz (75g) raw cane sugar
2 teaspoonsful dried pectin
6 oz (150g) ground brown rice
1 oz (25g) yellow split pea flour
4 oz (100g) ground almonds
1 slightly heaped tablespoonful special wheat-free and milk-free baking powder (see recipe, page 25)
3 heaped teaspoonsful cinnamon
3 tablespoonsful sunflower oil or similar
⅔ pint (350ml) unsweetened pineapple juice
6 oz (150g) finely grated eating apple
2 oz (50g) finely grated carrot
Rind of 1 lemon and 1 orange, coarsely grated
1 lb (½ kilo) dried fruit salad, washed well

American

½ cupful soy flour
½ cupful raw cane sugar
2 teaspoonsful dried pectin
¾ cupful ground brown rice
2½ tablespoonsful yellow split pea flour
1 cupful ground almonds
1 slightly heaped tablespoonful special wheat-free and milk-free baking soda (see recipe, page 25)
3 heaped teaspoonsful cinnamon
3 tablespoonsful sunflower oil or similar
1½ cupsful unsweetened pineapple juice
2 small eating apples, finely grated
1 small carrot, finely grated
Rind of 1 lemon and 1 orange, coarsely grated
2⅔ cupsful dried fruit salad, washed well

1. Preheat oven at 400°F/200°C (Gas Mark 6).

2. Put all the nine dry ingredients into a bowl and mix well.

3. Add the oil, orange juice, grated apple and carrot. Mix again.

4. Stir in the rinds and the fruit. (De-stone prunes.)

5. Oil and flour with ground brown rice an 8 in. (20cm) diameter cake tin (round). Spoon in the cake mix and flatten the top with a knife.

6. Bake near the top of the oven for about 1 hour.

7. Leave for a minute or two before turning out on to a wire rack to cool.

8. Use within 7 to 8 days and store in an air-tight container.

Note: This makes a lovely, moist rich fruit cake. Nobody will be able to tell the difference between this cake and an ordinary one so don't be afraid to hand it round!

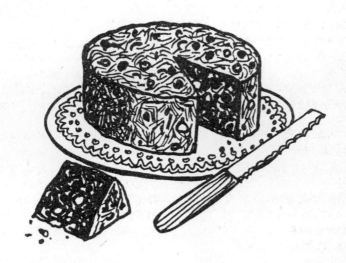

FRUIT, SPICE AND NUT CAKE

As well as being a festival cake this makes a sensible standby as it keeps for at least a week and is a moist and substantial wholefood, useful for people who find a diet without wheat tends to make them lose too much weight. It is also impressive and very similar to rich fruit cake made with wheat, eggs, etc. Just the kind of cake to make people envious of special diet food!

Imperial (Metric)	American
½ pint (¼ litre) orange juice	1⅓ cupsful orange juice
4 heaped tablespoonsful raw cane sugar	4 heaped tablespoonsful raw cane sugar
½ oz (15g) dried yeast granules	1 tablespoonful dried yeast granules
2 average eating apples	2 average eating apples
1 medium fresh carrot	1 medium fresh carrot
3 tablespoonsful sunflower oil	3 tablespoonsful sunflower oil

Flour Blend:

Imperial (Metric)	American
2 oz (50g) soya flour	½ cupful soy flour
9 oz (250g) brown ground rice	1¼ cupsful brown ground rice
1 oz (25g) yellow split pea flour	2 tablespoonsful yellow split pea flour
2 heaped teaspoonsful wheat-free mixed spice	2 heaped teaspoonsful wheat-free mixed spice
2 heaped teaspoonsful ground cinnamon	2 heaped teaspoonsful ground cinnamon
4 oz (100g) ground almonds	1 cupful ground almonds

Fruit:

Imperial (Metric)	American
1 lb (½ kilo) dried fruit — any mixture of raisins, sultanas, and currants	1 pound dried fruit — any mixture of golden seedless raisins and currants
4 oz (100g) chopped, dried apricots	1 cupful chopped, dried apricots
Coarsley grated rind of 1 orange and 1 lemon	Coarsley grated rind of 1 orange and 1 lemon

Decoration:

Imperial (Metric)	American
1 oz (25g) each of split almonds, walnut halves and hazelnuts	¼ cupful each of split almonds, English walnut halves and hazelnuts

1. Preheat oven at 350°F/180°C (Gas Mark 4).

2. Heat the fruit juice with the sugar until warm (not hot). Put into the liquidizer goblet and sprinkle in the dried yeast. Now leave to let the yeast soften while you blend the flour.

3. Put the flour ingredients into a large mixing bowl. Spoon in the oil and stir.

4. Chop the apple and carrot and add to the liquidizer. Blend and pour over the flour.

5. Stir well to a sloppy mixture and then add the fruit and rinds. Stir again.

6. Oil a large cake tin, approx 9 in. (23cm) diameter. Spoon the mixture into this and flatten the top.

7. Decorate with the nuts, pressing them slightly into the surface.

8. Bake in the top shelf for about an hour.

9. Leave in the tin to cool down. Cut when cold.

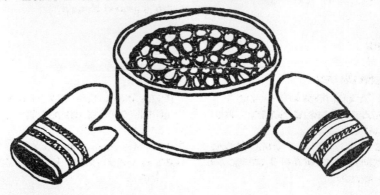

FRUIT 'CHEESECAKE'

Base:

Imperial (Metric)	American
4 oz (100g) any special biscuits made from a recipe in this book	4 ounces any special biscuits made from a recipe in this book
1½ oz (40g) milk-free margarine	3½ tablespoonsful milk-free margarine

1. Crush the biscuits into crumbs and put them into a basin.

2. Melt the margarine gently in a saucepan and pour it over the crumbs.

3. Mix well. Cut a piece of foil to fit the bottom of a sponge tin or a shallow, straight-sided dish.

4. Grease with milk-free margarine and spread the crumb mixture evenly over this.

Filling:

Imperial (Metric)	American
2 oz (50g) milk-free margarine	¼ cupful milk-free margarine
2 oz (50g) yellow split pea flour	½ cupful yellow split pea flour
½ lb (¼ kilo) cooked dried apricots, liquidized in ¼ pint (150ml) water	1½ cupsful cooked dried apricots, liquidized in ⅔ cupful water
1 tablespoonful lemon juice	1 tablespoonful lemon juice
Grated rind of 1 lemon	Grated rind of 1 lemon
2 pinches of cinnamon	2 pinches of cinnamon
1 heaped tablespoonful raw cane sugar	1 heaped tablespoonful raw cane sugar

1. Melt the margarine in a saucepan and add the split pea flour.

2. Fry for 2 to 3 minutes, stirring all the time.

3. Pour in the liquidized juice/water and all other ingredients. Stir well and cook for another 3 to 4 minutes until you have a stiff paste.

4. Cool a little and spread over the crumb base. Flatten with a knife and allow to cool.

Topping:
Cover with a generous layer of raw sugar jam (jelly) — any variety.

Note: Store in the fridge and eat within two days of making.

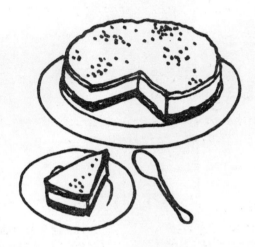

PEAR UPSIDE-DOWN CAKE

Topping:

Imperial (Metric)	American
Milk-free margarine	Milk-free margarine
2 oz (50g) raw cane sugar	1/3 cupful raw cane sugar
4 pears, peeled and halved	4 pears, peeled and halved

Base:

Imperial (Metric)	American
1 oz (25g) soya flour	1/4 cupful soy flour
2 oz (50g) raw cane sugar	1/3 cupful raw cane sugar
1 teaspoonful dried pectin	1 teaspoonful dried pectin
1 oz (25g) potato flour	2 1/2 tablespoonsful potato flour
4 oz (100g) ground brown rice	1/2 cupful ground brown rice
1 oz (25g) yellow split pea flour	2 1/2 tablespoonsful yellow split pea flour
1 oz (25g) ground almonds	1/4 cupful ground almonds
1 slightly heaped tablespoonful special baking powder (page 25)	1 slightly heaped tablespoonful special baking soda (page 25)
1/3 pint (200ml) unsweetened orange juice	3/4 cupful unsweetened orange juice
1 tablespoonful sunflower oil or similar	1 tablespoonful sunflower oil or similar
1 oz (25g) wheat-free cocoa	1/4 cupful wheat-free cocoa

1. Liberally grease a straight-sided, shallow round dish, about the size of a sponge tin. Sprinkle all over with the sugar and place the pears, cut side down and with the tops pointing in towards the centre of the dish.

2. Preheat oven at 400°F/200°C (Gas Mark 6).

3. Put all ingredients into a bowl and mix with a wooden spoon until you have a creamy cake mix.

4. Spread carefully over the pear halves and fill in the gaps.

5. Flatten with a knife and bake on the top shelf for about 30 minutes.

6. Leave to cool for 5 minutes and then cover with a plate.

7. Turn upside-down and lift the dish off carefully.

Variation: Omit cocoa and increase the potato flour by ½ oz (15g)/1½ tablespoonsful. Add ½ teaspoonful of cinnamon to the cake mix and use halved, stoned fresh apricots for the fruit. You will need about 7 or 8 fruits.

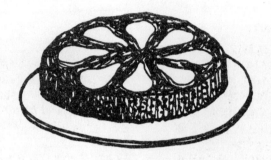

SWEET MINCEMEAT

Imperial (Metric)	American
3 oz (75g) sultanas	½ cupful golden seedless raisins
2 oz (50g) raisins	⅓ cupful raisins
3 oz (75g) currants	½ cupful carrots
2 oz (50g) raw cane sugar	⅓ cupful raw cane sugar
2 oz (50g) melted milk-free margarine	¼ cupful melted milk-free margarine
2 oz (50g) chopped walnuts and almonds mixed	½ cupful chopped English walnuts and almonds mixed
½ teaspoonful allspice	½ teaspoonful allspice
½ teaspoonful cinnamon	½ teaspoonful cinnamon
½ teaspoonful freshly grated nutmeg	½ teaspoonful freshly grated nutmeg
Finely grated rind of 1 lemon	Finely grated rind of 1 lemon
1 eating apple, grated	1 eating apple, grated
Orange juice, fresh	Orange juice, fresh

1. Blend all ingredients in a bowl and moisten with a little orange juice — about 2 tablespoonsful should be enough.

2. Store in covered jars in the fridge and use as required.

   This will keep for several weeks. As the commercial type of sweet mincemeat usually contains suet, which is rolled in wheat flour, home-made mincemeat will be the safest to use and is really much nicer than the bought kind.

MINCEMEAT TART

Use the recipe for Fruit Tart but use mincemeat instead of the fruit. Bake as directed.

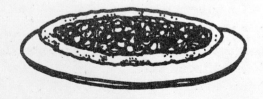

SESAME CRACKERS
(Makes about 12-15)

Imperial (Metric)
4 oz (100g) *Trufree* No. 6 plain flour
1 oz (25g) milk-free margarine
2 pinches of sea salt
Cold water to mix
Extra flour for rolling out etc.
Sesame seeds

American
½ cupful *Trufree* No. 6 plain flour
2½ tablespoonsful milk-free
 margarine
2 pinches of sea salt
Cold water to mix
Extra flour for rolling out etc.
Sesame seeds

1. Preheat oven at 450°F/230°C (Gas Mark 8).

2. Put the flour into a basin with the margarine and salt and rub in with the fingers until the mixture resembles fine breadcrumbs.

3. Add a little water (to release the binder in the flour) and mix to a stiff paste with a fork. Add more water if required.

5. Knead quickly into one lump of soft dough.

6. Roll out thinly and cut into squares or rectangles.

7. Use a spatula to place the pieces on ungreased baking sheets. Prick with a fork. Brush with water and sprinkle with sesame seeds.

8. Bake for about 8 to 10 minutes on the top shelf until golden but not brown.

9. Take off the baking sheets, leave to cool and crisp on a wire rack.

10. Store in an air-tight container.

Variation: Omit sesame seeds for plain water biscuits.

COCKTAIL BISCUITS
Make and bake as for Water Biscuits but cut into much smaller biscuits and bake for 2 or 3 minutes less.

SACRISTANS

Any of the pastry recipes suggested in this book are suitable. Use leftover pieces, before they are baked. Press together and roll out more thickly than usual. Brush with water and press in chopped plain nuts. Sprinkle with sea salt to taste. Cut into fingers and bake as for pastry.

APPLE CHUTNEY

Imperial (Metric)	American
1 lb (½ kilo) cooking apples, peeled and chopped	1 pound cooking apples, peeled and chopped
4 oz (100g) onions, peeled and chopped	1 cupful onions, peeled and chopped
3 oz (75g) sultanas	½ cupful golden seedless raisins
¼ pint (150ml) cider vinegar	⅔ cupful cider vinegar
2 oz (50g) raw cane sugar	⅓ cupful raw cane sugar
¼ teaspoonful ground ginger	¼ teaspoonful ground ginger
¼ teaspoonful sea salt	¼ teaspoonful sea salt

1. Cook the apple, onion, sultanas (golden seedless raisins) and dates in the vinegar until soft.

2. Add the remaining ingredients and stir well.

3. Bring to the boil and simmer until you have a thick chutney.

4. Put into clean, hot jars and allow to cool before covering.

5. Store in the fridge and use as required. (Serve with curry or cold meats.)

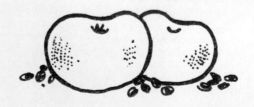

TOMATO KETCHUP

Imperial (Metric)
1 lb (½ kilo) ripe tomatoes
3 teaspoonsful Tarragon vinegar
3 tablespoonsful raw cane sugar
2 pinches each of cinnamon,
  cayenne pepper, sea salt, ground
  mace and allspice

American
1 pound ripe tomatoes
3 teaspoonsful Tarragon vinegar
3 tablespoonsful raw cane sugar
2 pinches each of cinnamon,
  cayenne pepper, sea salt, ground
  mace and allspice

1. Put the tomatoes into a pan, after slicing. Add a little water if required and cook for about 3 or 4 minutes, while stirring.

2. Allow to cool and liquidize.

3. Return to pan and add sugar and spices. Stir well.

4. Bring to the boil and simmer until it has reduced to a thick sauce.

5. Allow to grow cold and put into a sauce bottle or jar. Use as required. Best stored in the fridge.

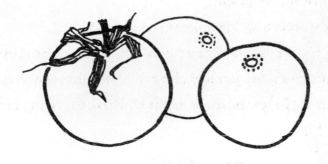

14.

MENUS BASED ON THE RECIPES IN THIS BOOK

Each day drink tea with lemon or black coffee, water or wine with your main meal if desired. Tea (food) is optional.

Day One
Breakfast — Savoury Breakfast Cakes.
Lunch — Mixed salad with a slice of cold beef or ham; Special Crispbread; fruit.
Tea — Fruit cake.
Dinner — Cauliflower Soup; Liver with Orange and Bacon, greens, root vegetables, mashed potato, gravy; Stuffed Baked Fruit.
Snacks — Fruit and nuts, banana.

Day Two
Breakfast — Beans on special toast, unsweetened fruit juice.
Lunch — Mixed green salad with tinned fish (in oil), mashed potato
Tea — Sultana Scones and special milk-free margarine.
Dinner — Avocado Soup; Pork Chop with Apple Salad, jacket potatoes with special milk-free margarine; Fruit Dessert.
Snacks — Ginger Thins, nuts.

Day Three
Breakfast — Small Muesli; grilled bacon and mushrooms.
Lunch — Lentil Soup, special bread (toasted) and milk-free margarine; Fruit Salad.
Tea — Dundee Cake.
Dinner — Liver Pâté with special toast; Prawns Italian with brown

rice, large green salad; Orange.

Snacks — Fruit and nuts, Digestive Biscuits.

Day Four

Breakfast — Kedgeree.

Lunch — Cold meat (chicken) and salad with mashed potato; fresh
fruit.

Tea — Fruit 'Cheesecake'.

Dinner — Beef Casserole with Orange, jacket potatoes, spinach or
greens; Baked Fruit.

Snacks — Crispbreads, special milk-free margarine and raw sugar
jam (jelly).

Day Five

Breakfast — Cold Meat and Fried Potatoes.

Lunch — Broad Bean Soup, Sippets; jacket potato with special milk-
free margarine.

Tea — Salad and mashed potato.

Dinner — Tomato Starter; Fish Casserole, green vegetables, boiled
brown rice; Stewed Fruit.

Snacks — Fresh fruit.

Day Six

Breakfast — Bubble and Squeak with grilled bacon.

Lunch — Fish and Chips.

Tea — Spiced Fruit Cookies.

Dinner — Grapefruit; Chicken Curry with brown rice and green salad;
Fresh Fruit or Fruit Salad.

Snacks — Bananas, nuts.

Day Seven

Breakfast — Savoury Breakfast Cakes.

Lunch — Cold fish, mixed salad, mashed potato; fruit.

Tea — Special toast, special milk-free margarine and raw sugar jam
(jelly).

Dinner — Lemon Chicken, boiled brown rice, stir-fry vegetables with

greens; Fruit Salad (with lychees if in season).
Snacks — Spiced Fruit Cookies.

Day Eight
Breakfast — Fruit Pancakes.
Lunch — Roast lamb, mint sauce, roast potatoes, green vegetables;
  Fried Bananas.
Tea — Special bread or Fruit Loaf and milk-free margarine; mixed
  salad with cold fish (tinned); special cake (from *Teas and Treats*
  section).
Snacks — Party Almonds, Special Cheese and Crispbreads.

Breakfasts
Savoury Breakfast Cakes with grilled tomatoes.
Small Muesli, grilled bacon and tomatoes.
Grilled bacon, tomatoes, fried mushrooms, special toast, milk-free
  margarine and raw sugar marmalade.
Breakfast Pizza.
Grilled fish, tomatoes and crispbreads with milk-free margarine.
Rice and Sultana Pudding, cold meat.
Grapefruit, slice of cold ham, tomato, special bread or crispbreads,
  milk-free margarine.
Fried potato and baked beans with mushrooms.
Baked beans on special toast with tomatoes.
Bubble and Squeak with grilled bacon, special toast, milk-free
  margarine and raw sugar marmalade.
Grapefruit with raw cane sugar, Kedgeree.
Savoury Breakfast Cakes, Fruit Pancake.
(Tea with lemon or black coffee, fruit juice, as required.)

Light Meals (suitable for lunch or high tea)
Fish Cakes with mixed salad.
Cold meat or fish with salad and mashed potato.
Liver and Mushroom Pâté on special toast with green salad.
French Country Soup with Sippets, Fruit Tart with Nuts.
Lentil Soup, jacket potato stuffed with chopped grilled bacon and
  mushrooms.

Shepherd's Pie with peas and grilled tomatoes.
Fish and chips with peas or grilled tomatoes.

Main Meals

Prawns Italian with green salad, plain boiled brown rice.
Lemon Chicken, plain boiled brown rice, green salad or stir-fry vegetables with plenty of green leaves.
Shepherd's Pie, carrots, peas, cabbage or sprouts.
Liver Provençale with plain boiled brown rice or mashed potatoes, green vegetables.
Goulash with plain boiled brown rice, green salad.
Roast beef or lamb (joint) with roast potatoes, green vegetables in season, gravy.
Pork Chop with Apple Salad, jacket potato.
Trout with Almonds, peas or a mixed salad.
Grilled Fish with Herbs, peas and carrots.
Lamb with Garlic and Rosemary (chops), roast potatoes and parsnip, greens.
Kebabs with plain boiled brown rice, green salad.
Baked Trout with mashed potato, grilled tomatoes, peas.
Grilled Steak with spinach, carrots and grilled tomatoes or Savoury Rice.
Grilled lamb chops (plain) with Savoury Rice.
Chicken Curry with plain boiled brown rice, sliced cucumber and tomato.
Chicken and Herb Casserole, mashed or jacket potato, green vegetables.
Beef Casserole with Orange, stir-fry vegetables.
Good, Old Fashioned Stew with green vegetables.
Lemon Chicken and Chinese Fried Rice, stir-fry vegetables.
Bolognaise Sauce with plain boiled brown rice, green salad.
Nut Roast, green vegetables, mashed potato.

Combine any of these main meals with a recipe from the puddings section to make a substantial meal. Really hearty eaters will enjoy something from the section which contains soups and starters too.

Teas

The bread-and-butter and cake teas our grandparents enjoyed have largely gone out of fashion. However, youngsters often go through a stage of always feeling hungry, usually when they are growing very quickly (early teens) and this can be a useful way of giving them an extra meal without too much trouble.

Sultana Scones with milk-free margarine, slice of fruit cake (from *Teas and Treats* section), apple.

Slices of Brown Tea Bread with milk-free margarine, fruit cake (from *Teas and Treats* section), banana

Special toast, milk-free margarine and raw sugar jam (jelly), Pear Upside-down Cake, nuts.

Sultana Scones or Crispbreads and milk-free margarine, Fruit 'Cheesecake'.

Soup with Sippets, fruit cake (from *Teas and Starters* section).

A good time to use up any kind of pudding left from the previous day.

Treats

It is amazing how many people believe that a 'treat' to someone on a special diet means the very things they are normally not allowed to eat, forgetting that these things will probably cause that person to be ill. The majority of people think that diets are merely for slimming and many are under the illusion that any kind of special diet is just a silly fad.

A treat should be either a special dish or food that is not a normal part of the diet, either because it requires some trouble to make or is expensive. It can also be something seasonal such as mince pies or Christmas Cake. Whatever form it takes it should still be firmly within the confines of the permitted foods on the diet. (See the index for suggestions.)

USEFUL INFORMATION

General Items
Available at most supermarkets or grocery stores:
Ground rice
Spices
Vegetable cooking oils
Dried yeast
Fruit juices
Wine or cider vinegar

Specialized Items
Probably available at health stores, delicatessens or large chemists
    (drugstores):
Soya flour
Potato flour (farina)
Maize flour (cornmeal)
Rice bran
Yellow split pea flour
Trufree (wheat-free) flours

Other Specialized Items
(guaranteed wheat-free, milk-free and egg-free)
If these ingredients are not available as suggested above, the
Cantassium Co. have a mail order service for people on special diets:
Pectin
Special baking powder
Yellow split pea flour

Ground brown rice
Rice bran
Potato flour (farina)
Maize flour (cornmeal)
Trufree vitamins and minerals
Trufree flours and *Trufree Crispbran* etc.

Write to: Dept WMEF, Cantassium Co., 225 Putney Bridge Road, London SW15 2PY.

Some small independent bakers sell baked *Trufree* breads etc. They are usually very helpful if you need regular supplies and some will bake special items for customers. Some will also supply hospitals in bulk (UK).

This book can also be used for gluten-free cooking if the four following points are considered:-

1. **Do not use oats or oatmeal.**
2. **Do not use bought crispbreads.**
3. **Use a soya sauce which is gluten-free.**
4. **Use gluten-free breakfast cereals.**

There is now a wheat-free sign to help you. Look for it on packets.

INDEX